Drugs and Clients

What Every Psychotherapist
Needs to Know

Padma Catell

Solarium Press

Petaluma, California

Published in the United States by Solarium Press,
an imprint of Castalia Communications, Petaluma, California

www.drugsandclients.com

Library of Congress Cataloging-in-Publication Data

Catell, Padma, 1944–
    Drugs and clients : what every psychotherapist needs to know / Padma Catell.-- 1st ed.
        p. cm.
    Includes bibliographical references and index.
            ISBN 0-929150-76-7 (trade pbk.) — ISBN 0-929150-75-9 (hardcover)
    1. Psychopharmacology. 2. Mental illness--Chemotherapy.
    3. Mentally ill—Substance abuse. I. Title.
RC483.C38 2004
615'.78–dc22   2004004743

Credits and Permissions:

Illustrations:
Kelli Bullock: Cover, pps. 18, 42, 74, 146
Padma Catell: pps. 64, 87, 110, 155, 159, 165
Edvard Munch: "The Scream" (1893) p. 94
Sir John Tenniel, from *Alice in Wonderland* (1865) p. 126
Unknown artists: pps. 1, 32

Editing and design: Scott Morrison
Indexing: Celeste Newbrough
Computer graphics: Jack Nau, Jerry Moffitt

Song lyric:
"Java Jive," by Ben Oakland & Milton Drake
© 1940 (Renewed) WB Music Corp. and Sony Tunes, Inc.
All Rights Reserved   Used by Permission
WARNER BROS. PUBLICATIONS U.S. INC. Miami, FL. 33014

Zoloft® is a Registered Trademark of the Pfizer Corporation.

Manufactured in the United States of America

This book is dedicated to the memory
of my two greatest teachers,
my mother, Belle Diamond,
and Sri Brahamananda Saraswati,
who told me I would write this book
years before I ever dreamed of it.

Acknowledgements

Over the years it has taken me to write this book there have been many people who have given me help and support. It is important for me to acknowledge some to whom I am particularly grateful.

I would like to start with Ralph Metzner, dear friend and fellow traveler, since he was the one who convinced me that I could teach psychopharmacology, and it was through the process of teaching that this volume was born.

I greatly appreciate the constant love I have received from my close friends, in particular Tanya Wilkinson, Rob Hopcke, and Paul Schwartz. Without them as a base, I would have floundered in the many trials of life.

I would like to thank the NOMAD dancers and the "tappers" who have brought joy to my heart through dance, regardless of the pain in the other parts of my life.

There are two living sages I seek out in times of dire confusion, Michael Kahn and Dean Elias, whose wisdom and kindness have been given with generosity whenever I have needed it.

I am grateful for my brother Bob, who has been quietly behind me as a source of support throughout my life. His love and generosity are appreciated by many, but I am the only one who has the good fortune to be able to claim him as my brother.

And finally, I want to thank my husband Scott, whose love, humor, and constancy have given me more than he can know, and without whom this book would truly never have been possible.

Contents

Tables & Figures

Author's Preface

I wrote this book primarily for practitioners trained in the art of psychotherapy, especially psychologists, Marriage and Family Therapists, and Clinical Social Workers, most of whom are not familiar with the biochemistry of psychotropic drugs and medications. I also wanted a textbook for use in my own course, Psychopharmacology for Psychotherapists, as I could not find a book in this field that specifically addressed the needs of today's psychology and counseling graduate students.

In recent years the vast increase in the use of psychoactive drugs, both legal and illegal, has made an understanding of how psychotropic substances affect clients far more important for psychotherapists than it has been in the past. It is vital that therapists have the ability to discuss the pros and cons of taking medication with their clients in a knowledgeable and unbiased way. Equally important for therapists is the ability to recognize the signs of adverse effects of prescription and non-prescription drugs as well as symptoms of substance abuse, physical dependency, and withdrawal.

It is my hope that this book will also prove to be useful to the many health and mental-health professionals who are not trained in the specialty of psychiatry but who work with clients who may be taking psychoactive medications or using nonprescription psychotropic drugs. I believe that the information which is presented here will contribute to attaining the ideal that all health-care professionals strive to achieve, the optimal treatment of all clients.

Padma Catell, Ph.D.
June, 2004

IMPORTANT NOTICE

This book is not to be used as a guide to prescribing, taking, or discontinuing any medication, vitamin, herbal preparation, aromatherapy product, food supplement or any other substance discussed, or not discussed, herein.

Any decision as to whether to prescribe, use, or administer anything discussed or not discussed in this book must first be evaluated by a licensed, and appropriately trained, medical practitioner.

No liability will be incurred by the author or the publisher for any errors or omissions, or for any actions, either taken or not taken, by anyone regarding the material included, or not included, in this volume.

Chapter 1
Sleep & Treatment of Sleep Disorders

The complex process of sleep is a universal human phenomenon that both affects and reflects our psychological and physical states in profound ways. Even though its specific function and purpose is not yet well-understood, the practicing psychotherapist should include an evaluation of a client's sleep problems and sleep patterns as a routine part of a comprehensive psychological assessment.

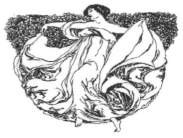

It has long been known that change in sleep patterns can be used as indicators for diagnosing anxiety and depression.[1,2] Some researchers believe that sleep disturbances may even cause these psychological disorders.[3] Many psychoactive drugs cause changes in "sleep architecture" (the stages of sleep and the length of time spent in each stage) (see Fig. 1.1).[4,5] In the last few years, there have been significant advances in understanding that sleep disturbances are an indication of fundamental alterations in functions of the *central nervous system* (CNS).

As many as one in three adults in the U.S. occasionally suffers from insomnia, and 10% to 15% suffer from it continually.[6] The insomnia frequently lasts for days and can sometimes last for weeks. Stress, depression, anxiety, and many drugs, dramatically affect our ability to sleep. Sleep problems have a very serious impact on society. The National Highway Traffic Safety Administration estimates that over 100,000 accidents every year are caused by drowsy drivers.[6] Although the specific role of sleep in health maintenance is still not clear, there is no doubt that lack of sleep can be detrimental to one's health. One large study[7] showed that people who slept fewer than five hours per night had a 30% higher rate of heart disease than those who slept more than five hours. The research demonstrated that older adults who had periods of wakefulness of 30 minutes or more during the night had decreased longevity compared with their better-rested peers. Seniors who had sleeplessness or extremely high or low amounts of REM sleep were about twice as likely to have died by the follow-up date (13 years later). Researchers are continuing to examine how treating older adults for sleep problems affects longevity.[7]

A connection between sleep and depression can be seen when patients are intentionally deprived of *rapid-eye-movement* (REM) sleep, the stage when most dreaming takes place. Depressive symptoms are alleviated by one night of sleep deprivation and recur after sleeping.[8] The vast majority of antidepressant medications suppress REM sleep, and evidence suggests that the mechanism of action for most antidepressants is somehow connected to the suppression of REM sleep.[4, 5] Though the details of the relationship between mental disorders and sleep are not yet understood, it is clear that a strong connection exists. A better understanding of this relationship could lead to new treatments for both psychological problems and sleep disorders.

Normal Sleep & the Sleep Cycle

To understand sleep disorders, it is important to understand the patterns of the normal sleep cycle (see Fig. 1.1).[3, 6, 9-11] It takes an average of 30 to 45 minutes after falling asleep to progress from Stage 1 to Delta. One then passes back from Delta to Stage 1. At this point, the first period of REM sleep usually occurs. For most people, REM begins approximately 90 minutes after falling asleep.[3] The period between falling asleep and the first onset of REM is termed *REM latency*.[11, 12] The duration of REM latency can be useful as a diagnostic measure for depressive, sleep, and anxiety disorders.

The percentage of time spent in REM sleep declines with age. REM takes up about 80% of life for an infant who is born prematurely, and about 50% for a full-term newborn. Young and middle-aged adults spend 20% of their sleep in REM, and the elderly only 15%.[12]

Most dreaming takes place during REM, and some dreaming occurs during Delta. We usually do not remember dreams that take place during Delta. When awakened from REM, people can recall dreams about 80% of the time. As sleep progresses through the night the periods of REM become more frequent, each episode of REM is longer, and the time between REM episodes decreases.[13]

The EEG becomes increasingly slower and more synchronized as one progresses from Stage 1 to Delta sleep. During Delta, the *parasympathetic nervous system* (PSNS), which controls homeostatic functions, dominates. There is an increase in gastrointestinal (GI) motility (movement), large muscles are relaxed (although there are some small body movements), heart rate slows, blood pressure decreases, and respiration rate slows and becomes more even.[13]

The phenomena of sleepwalking and *night terrors* (when children scream in their sleep and seem to be having terrifying dreams from which it is difficult to awaken them) both occur during Delta sleep. The length of time spent in each period of Delta becomes shorter as the night progresses. For most people, sleep becomes "lighter" toward the end of the sleep cycle, and awakenings are more frequent.[13] Although this sleep pattern is the norm, there are many individual

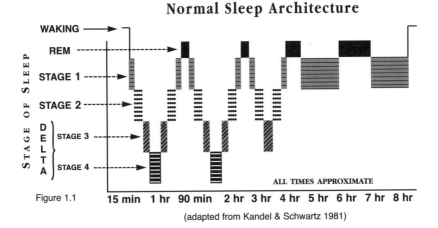

Normal Sleep Architecture

Figure 1.1

ALL TIMES APPROXIMATE

15 min   1 hr   90 min   2 hr   3 hr   4 hr   5 hr   6 hr   7 hr   8 hr

(adapted from Kandel & Schwartz 1981)

differences. Some people report that they sleep more deeply toward morning.

Delta sleep may disappear completely in people over age 60.[3] This progressive decrease in Delta contributes to the increase in insomnia and the many spontaneous awakenings experienced by the elderly.

Stages of Sleep

The stages of sleep are primarily defined by changes in EEG patterns. Body movements and eye movements may also be specific to the various sleep stages.

Sleep latency

This is the period between lying down and closing one's eyes, and the start of Stage 1 sleep (on average about 10 to 15 minutes).[12]

Stage 1

The initial stage of sleep is relatively brief, usually between 30 seconds and 7 minutes. Reactivity to outside stimuli is diminished, thoughts begin to drift, and short dreams may take place. The EEG will indicate brain waves in the theta range, which is between three and seven cycles per second (cps).[12]

Stage 2

During this stage mental processes consist of short, fragmented thoughts. Stage 2 is marked by the appearance on the EEG of a pattern known as "sleep spindles." These denote bursts of brain activity in the 12 to 14 cps range, each lasting between one-half and two seconds, This stage occurs repeatedly throughout the night.[12]

Delta

Delta is the "deepest" stage of sleep and combines what were historically known as Stage 3 and Stage 4 sleep. This stage is distinguished by the presence of delta waves on the EEG. Delta waves are one-half to two cps and have high amplitudes. This slow-frequency, high-amplitude pattern must exist in at least 20% of the EEG to be designated as Delta sleep. It is difficult to be awakened from Delta sleep. The percentage of time spent in Delta decreases with age. Research has shown that by the time men reach the age of 45, they have nearly lost their ability to fall into deep sleep.[12]

Rapid-eye movement (REM)

REM sleep resembles Stage 1 in its EEG pattern. During REM, the EEG becomes desynchronized and shows waves of higher frequency and lower voltage than in the other stages of sleep. EEG patterns are similar to the wakeful state. REM sleep can be further separated into *tonic* and *phasic* components; these are physiologically distinct from each other. Tonic REM is characterized by muscle paralysis in skeletal muscles, increased cerebral blood flow, and an increase in brain temperature. Phasic REM includes short episodes of rapid-eye movement and muscle twitching; the body seems highly activated. REM sleep is when most dreaming takes place. This closeness to the waking state facilitates the ability to remember dreams. Contrary to popular belief, REM is not a "deep" stage of sleep. One can easily be awakened during REM sleep.[12]

Effects of Drugs on Sleep Architecture

Benzodiazepines (BZs)

Delta sleep is reduced by benzodiazepines (e.g., diazepam/Valium, alprazolam/Xanax) much more than is REM sleep. This reduction in Delta leads to a decrease in night terrors and some nightmares. BZs are used to treat these disorders since they decrease, and eventually eliminate, deep sleep.[4]

Selective serotonin reuptake inhibitors (SSRIs)

Research shows that because it reduces deep sleep, the

antidepressant paroxetine/Paxil (and probably all the SSRIs) can be helpful in treatment of night terrors.[4]

Alcohol & barbiturates

Chronic use of both alcohol and barbiturates causes a suppression of REM sleep. Barbiturate use leads to an increase in Stage 2 and a decrease in Delta sleep.[13] People with a history of drug or alcohol abuse may experience sleep disturbances for many years after cessation of the drug or alcohol use. Problems with falling asleep and a decrease in Delta sleep are frequently seen during abstinence after habitual use. Gabapentin/Neurontin has been found to be the best treatment for this insomnia.[14] The specific reason or reasons for the long-term disturbance of sleep is unclear. (See Fig.2.1.)

REM rebound

REM rebound is the increase in time spent in REM sleep following a period of REM deprivation.[3] Most likely it is the body's attempt to compensate for the loss. The duration varies from person to person, and is related to the extent of the deprivation. REM rebound is marked by an increase in the number of spontaneous awakenings during the night and by an increase in restlessness and dreaming. A person may feel sleep deprived during REM rebound due to the corresponding decrease in Delta sleep. No serious mental problems seem to be caused by REM sleep deprivation.

Neurotransmitters & Neuromodulators in Sleep

Wakefulness and sleep are discrete processes mediated by different substances in the central nervous system.[9,15] Many drugs, by affecting specific *neurotransmitters* (NTs) and *neuromodulators* (NMs), cause changes in sleep patterns. These NTs and NMs, in addition to their involvement in sleep and wakefulness, have a role in a wide variety of processes in the CNS, including mental and emotional states.

Serotonin (5-HT, 5-hydroxytryptamine)

Serotonin (abbreviated 5-HT) seems to be the neuromodulator most "involved" in sleep induction. Taking 5-HT precursors (in particular the amino acid tryptophan) leads to an increase in 5-HT synthesis, which facilitates the ability to fall asleep.[13]

Norepinephrine (NE)

The presence of norepinephrine (abbreviated NE) seems to be related to alertness and symptoms of anxiety. It is known to have a role in the symptoms of depression.[13]

Dopamine (DA)

Dopamine (abbreviated DA) is involved in reward processes, pleasurable states, and normal movement. DA seems to facilitate stimulation of reward centers in the CNS.[16]

Hypocretin-1 & hypocretin-2 (orexins)

These chemicals are found in the hypothalamic center in the CNS, which regulates sleep and the endocrine system. It is postulated that hypocretin is necessary to maintain a non-REM state. Levels of these substances are low in humans with narcolepsy, and completely absent in the narcoleptic dogs used in studies of sleep disorders.[17, 18]

Acetylcholine (ACh)

This neurotransmitter (abbreviated ACh) has a role in REM and Delta sleep, movement, and cognition. Experiments show that the firing of ACh neurons increases during Delta, and increases even more during REM.[3]

Sleep Disorders

Disorders of initiating & maintaining sleep

Sleep problems are frequently seen in conjunction with affective, personality, and somatoform (involving the body) disorders. Treatment for these may include analytic psychotherapy and behavioral therapy, either alone, or in combination with psychoactive compounds such as sedative, *anxiolytic* (anxiety decreasing), antidepressant, and antimanic medications (see Chapters 2, 4, and 5 for detailed discussions of these compounds). There are many medical disorders in this category.

Alternative treatments for insomnia

Many alternative treatments for insomnia are currently being tried. Some nutritional supplements are known to aid sleep:

- Calcium: For adults, 600 mg before bed
- Magnesium: 250 mg taken at bedtime
- Vitamin B_6:   50 to 100 mg daily may prevent insomnia
- Vitamin B_{12}:   25 mg supplemented with 100 mg of vitamin B_5 can serve as an effective anti-insomnia regimen[17]

(See Chapter 11 for more information on herbal and aromatherapy treatments for insomnia.)

Disorders of excessive somnolence

People who suffer from these disorders have the experience of getting lots of sleep, yet they always feel sleepy.[12]

NARCOLEPSY

Narcolepsy is due to abnormal occurrences of REM sleep. Symptoms of narcolepsy, such as taking frequent naps and excessive sleepiness, can easily be misdiagnosed as a lack of motivation or as depression. Between 50,000 and 250,000 people in the United States suffer from narcolepsy. Males and females are affected equally. There is strong evidence that narcolepsy has a genetic component; the relatives of narcoleptics are much more likely to develop the disorder than the average person.[3]

Most sleep researchers believe that narcolepsy is greatly under-diagnosed.[6] A definitive diagnosis usually requires spending one to three nights in a sleep laboratory for brain-wave (electroencephalo-gram/EEG) pattern monitoring during sleep.[3] These diagnostic procedures are expensive, and sleep laboratories are still scarce. Both of these factors contribute to the under-diagnosis of narcolepsy.

A person with narcolepsy goes directly into REM sleep rather than progressing through the other stages of sleep before going into the first REM period; this would normally take about 90 minutes.[11] (See Fig. 1.1). Going directly into REM causes the symptoms of *cataplexy*, sleep paralysis, and hypnogogic hallucinations.

Recognizing the symptoms of narcolepsy is important for the psychotherapist because these symptoms can be confused with depression, and because psychoactive medication is usually a component of the treatment. When narcolepsy is suspected, referral to a psychiatrist for a diagnosis and a medication evaluation is always necessary.

Etiology of narcolepsy

Narcolepsy is believed to be an inherited neurological disorder that shows itself as an abnormally high incidence of REM sleep. Researchers have discovered a specific neurotransmitter, hypocretin, which seems to be necessary to keep one awake. Hypocretin is produced primarily by cells in the *hypothalamus*. These cells are missing or damaged in people with narcolepsy. There is evidence that the damage may be due to an autoimmune reaction.[18-20]

Symptoms of narcolepsy

Everyone occasionally experiences some of the symptoms of narcolepsy. For a diagnosis of narcolepsy, at least four of the symptoms, or the presence of cataplexy, is required. Even when many symptoms are present, analysis by a sleep expert is essential for a definitive diagnosis.[3]

Symptoms usually begin between the ages of 10 and 20, and the disorder typically lasts for life. Symptoms generally reach a plateau in severity and then remain constant. Many patients report that they gain better control over their symptoms as they get older.[6] Usually, the first two symptoms experienced are *sleep attacks* and *excessive daytime sleepiness* (EDS).[3] Cataplexy may develop early in the disease, simultaneously with sleep attacks and daytime sleepiness, though in some people cataplexy does not appear until many years after the initial symptoms.[3]

Excessive daytime sleepiness (EDS)

Excessive daytime sleepiness affects approximately 250,000 Americans every year. This symptom usually develops over a period of several years. Usually the first symptoms of EDS are an increase in sleepiness and sleep attacks (see below).[3] EDS can be experienced either by itself or as a symptom of narcolepsy or other disorders. EDS indicates actual sleepiness (as differentiated from fatigue, depression, or lack of energy). An EDS sufferer has sudden, irresistible episodes of sleepiness, often at highly inappropriate times, such as when driving, eating, or having sex. Episodes occur on an almost daily basis. On average, someone with EDS takes only five minutes to fall asleep, compared with ten minutes or more for most people.[12]

Symptoms of EDS usually indicate a serious organic disorder, generally either narcolepsy or sleep apnea. There are many psychological conditions, such as depression, which may have fatigue as a symptom. Until recently, an accurate diagnosis for EDS required a costly night or two in a sleep lab. New technology has been developed which may facilitate many more accurate diagnoses. Patients can sleep at home while connected to recorders with later evaluation of the recordings by a sleep expert.[3]

Sleep attacks

Sleep attacks are the tendency to fall asleep in situations in which many people might feel sleepy, such as after a meal, or while listening to a boring speaker. These attacks are a manifestation of going directly into REM without first passing through the other stages of sleep.[3]

With narcolepsy, sleep attacks increase in frequency and begin to occur in situations that are less usual for people who are not affected by this disorder, such as while reading a newspaper, writing a letter, or waiting in line at a store. After a while, a person who has narcolepsy begins to fall asleep at times that are less appropriate, such as while driving a car or even in the middle of a conversation.

Each sleep attack can last from a few seconds to about 15 minutes. Often, the person may not realize he or she has been asleep and may behave oddly upon awakening, such as continuing a conversation or activity exactly where it left off.[3] During a sleep attack, a dream may be perceived as a real event because the person has is no internal awareness of the period of sleep. The experience can be very confusing, both for the person with narcolepsy and for anyone else who happens to be nearby.

Priamipexole/Mirapex and ropinerole/Requip, two drugs used to treat Parkinson's disease, have been found to cause sleep attacks.[13] Sleep attacks brought on by these drugs have occurred while patients were driving and have resulted in accidents. Because it is impossible to predict which patients on these drugs are most likely to experience sleep attacks, it is recommended that users of these medications not drive. The attacks cease when the drugs are discontinued.

Cataplexy

Cataplexy is a short episode, usually lasting a few seconds to 30 minutes, in which there is a decrease—or even a complete loss—of voluntary muscle control. This symptom is caused by going directly into REM sleep and the corresponding muscle paralysis that occurs during REM. Severity ranges from slight feelings of muscle weakness to a state of collapse that involves all voluntary muscles.[3]

Cataplectic attacks can be brought on by emotion, stress, or fatigue. The most frequent cause is strong emotion, in particular laughter and anger. An attack can be triggered by a stimulus as minor as the memory of an emotional situation. At first, cataplectic attacks are usually mild and infrequent; they generally progress in severity and frequency and reach a plateau. The intensity of the episodes may vary from one attack to the next. The frequency of the attacks differs from person to person, and may range from one or two per year to hundreds of attacks each day. A cataplectic attack may develop into a sleep attack if the person is reclining or sitting. The sufferer remains aware of his or her surroundings; this differentiates cataplexy from a seizure. The presence of cataplexy in narcolepsy ranges from 65% to 90%. Cataplexy is a definitive indicator for a diagnosis of narcolepsy.[3]

Automatic behavior

Automatic behavior is when a person does something and subsequently has no conscious recollection of having done it (e.g., driving somewhere and having no memory of how one got there, or putting dirty dishes in the clothes dryer and being awakened by the sound of breaking dishes). To a casual observer automatic behavior may not seem noteworthy or appear any different from normal activity. People suffering from it may be aware of a blank space in their memory during these periods. This symptom can be a source of confusion or shame, particularly if it is not recognized as caused by narcolepsy.[3]

Sleep paralysis

Sleep paralysis is an inability to move which usually occurs when falling asleep or shortly before waking up. Common feelings are not being able to open one's eyes, speak, or run away. The experience is generally uncomfortable and frightening. It is often described as feeling paralyzed coupled with the fear that there is a menacing figure nearby intent on doing one harm. There is usually complete recall of the episode after waking. Sleep paralysis is a common experience for many people who do not have narcolepsy or any other disorder.[3]

Hypnogogic hallucinations

Hypnogogic hallucinations are vivid, brief dreams that occur when falling asleep.[3] There is sometimes difficulty distinguishing these hallucinations from the waking state.

Sleep apnea with narcolepsy

People with narcolepsy often have other sleep disorders. About 20% of male narcoleptic patients also have sleep apnea.[6] (See below).

Treatment of narcolepsy

Although there is currently no cure for narcolepsy, the symptoms can be somewhat controlled with psychoactive medications. Stimulants such as amphetamines/Adderall, methylphenidate/Ritalin, or a drug called modafinil/Provigil, may decrease excessive sleepiness.[20] Modafinil is unique in that it does not stimulate brain centers to cause euphoria and is not considered a stimulant. It is in a class of drugs called *somnolytics*.[3, 21]

Since antidepressant medications suppress REM sleep, they can be used to treat attacks of cataplexy, sleep paralysis, and hypnogogic hallucinations.[5] Taking naps during the day and avoiding alcohol and other CNS depressants can also be helpful in alleviating symptoms. Sodium oxybate/Xyrem has recently been approved for the treatment of cataplexy.[22] It is believed to consolidate sleep, reduce cataplectic attacks, and reduce the severity of EDS.

REM SLEEP BEHAVIOR DISORDER

This disorder is the result of a breakdown in the brain process that prevents motor activity during REM sleep (phasic REM). This breakdown allows the movement of large muscles during dreaming.

The usual symptoms are kicking, punching, arm-swinging, and other movements that seem to be the acting out of dreams.

Over 90% of those affected with REM behavior disorder are men over the age of 50. There is some evidence that it is associated with narcolepsy, Parkinson's disease, Lewy body disease, and multiple-system atrophy. It has been found to occur in animals when cells in the area of the CNS called the pons are lesioned. There is evidence this disorder may be the first sign of the depletion of dopamine that later leads to Parkinson's disease. Clonazepam (a BZ which interferes with REM sleep) is used to decrease the symptoms of REM behavior disorder.[3]

SLEEP APNEA

Sleep apnea is a common cause of disrupted sleep and affects about 4% of men and 2% of women.[11] The apnea is a suspension of breathing that can last from 10 to 120 seconds, and is marked by heavy snoring and a struggle to breathe. It occurs when the upper airway collapses repeatedly during sleep. After a while, the person becomes semi-awake and breathing resumes. More than 75 awakenings per night are required for a diagnosis of apnea (some people experience hundreds of episodes during a single night).

A sufferer may have no specific awareness of the apnea, but the next day may feel excessively sleepy, have difficulty concentrating, and have no idea as to the cause. Frequently, it is the partner of someone with apnea who notices something is wrong, becomes frightened by the irregular breathing or gasping during the night, and requests that their partner be evaluated by a physician.

Because of their sleep-deprived state, those with apnea are six times more likely to have traffic accidents. Often life-style changes, like losing weight, quitting smoking, and avoiding alcohol and/or sleeping pills will decrease the episodes. This type of apnea is effectively treated with a device that provides *continuous positive air pressure* (CPAP) or with laser surgery to open up the airway.[3]

Direct Relevance to Psychotherapy

Feeling rested contributes to a state of psychological and physical well-being. Psychotherapists need to inquire about their clients' sleep habits and assess for possible problems. Even in so-called "normal" aging there is an increase in sleep difficulties. People often do not realize that anxiety and depression affect sleep patterns, so they do not report difficulties or changes in sleep to their therapists. Many clients may not mention that they are taking some form of sleep aid on a daily or as-needed basis. Clients may consume a wide range of products reputed to aid in falling asleep or staying asleep, including herbal teas, over-the-counter sleep medications, prescription sedatives or antianxiety drugs, the hormone melatonin, the amino acid tryptophan, and others. Many people are dependent on some type of sleep aid to obtain what they think of as "a good night's sleep."

The psychotherapist needs to assess the client's level of knowledge about normal sleep patterns and whether there is an understanding of the changes that take place with age. The psychotherapist can also gather information as to whether medications are being taken that might affect a client's sleep patterns and give feedback about this to both the client and to the prescribing psychiatrist. The psychotherapist is usually in the best position to synthesize all the pieces of information and consult with the client and the psychiatrist to determine what can be done to help the client achieve a more restful night's sleep and a better understanding of the sleep process.[23]

Appropriate treatment always depends upon accurate diagnosis. Interventions need to consider underlying disorders rather than just symptoms. If the underlying disorder is treated successfully, the sleep problem is usually alleviated. An accurate diagnosis is particularly critical if medication is to be a component of the client's treatment. Without a complete psychological assessment, treating the sleep disorder with medication can worsen both the sleep disorder and the psychological condition.

In general, anxiety is correlated with difficulty falling asleep, whereas depression is correlated with early morning awakening. If difficulty falling asleep is due to an underlying anxiety disorder, treatment with antianxiety medications might be the most appropriate pharmacological intervention.[4] (See Chapter 2.)

About 70% of patients with insomnia have depression as the underlying cause. The remaining 30% have other sleep disorders. If the sleep problem is caused by depression, then taking BZs (see Table 2.1) may actually worsen the depression, and over time can increase sleep difficulties.[6] Treatment with an antidepressant would be a more appropriate intervention in these cases.

The use of sleep medication every night is not recommended. Certain BZs classified as *hypnotics* (triazolam, flurazepam, temazepam) are helpful with sleep problems if taken for less than two weeks, or if not used more than three nights in a row. If taken longer or more frequently, sleep architecture will be altered.[5]

When psychotic symptoms are present, a specific diagnosis is critical before medications are chosen. An acute psychotic episode is often accompanied by sleep problems. The presence of hallucinations, feelings of persecution, and other fears, can frequently lead to sleep disturbances. Psychological treatments and medications used to alleviate symptoms differ greatly depending upon whether the underlying cause of the sleep problem is a psychosis, depression, or anxiety.

There may also be sleep disturbances with no underlying psychological problem. Due to individual sleep rhythms, one person may not be able to sleep during the night, then falls asleep in the early morning, and sleeps until mid-day. These patterns can be relatively easy to modify; if this is the cause of the difficulty, the most appropriate treatment may be education in techniques of basic sleep hygiene. Many books are available on this topic.[23, 24]

It is very common for a client to have some type of sleep disorder along with various psychological problems. A client may be taking medication for either the sleep disorder or the psychological disorder. For optimal treatment, it is important for the psychotherapist to consult with the prescribing psychiatrist whenever a client is on psychoactive medications and a sleep disorder is a presenting problem.

References for Chapter 1

1. Perlis, M. L., Giles, D. E., Buysse, D. J., Tu, X. & Kupfer, D. J. (1997). Self-reported sleep disturbance as a prodromal symptom in recurrent depression. *J. Affective Disorders*, 42(2–3), 209–212.

2. Lamb, M. (2000). Is it just insomnia? *Psychology Today*, March/April, 14.

3. Dement, W. C. & Vaughan, C. (1999). *The promise of sleep: A pioneer in sleep medicine explores the vital connection between health, happiness, and a good night's sleep.* New York, NY: Delacorte Press.

4. Armitage, R., Yonkers, K., Cole, D. & Rush, J. (1997). A multicenter, double-blind comparison of the effects of nefazodone and fluoxetine on sleep architecture and quality of sleep in depressed outpatients. *J. Clinical Psychopharm.*, 17(3), 161–168.

5. Vogel, G. W., Buffenstein, A., Minter, K. & Hennessey, A. (1990). Drug effects on REM sleep and on endogenous depression. *Neuropsy. Biobehav. Review*, 14, 49–63.

6. National Sleep Foundation. 888-NSF-SLEEP. Retrieved from http://www.sleepfoundation.org/ Information on sleep disorders and sleep disorder clinics.

7. Dew, M. A., PhD, Hoch, C. C., Buysse, D. J., Monk, T. H., Begley, A. E., Houck, P. R., Hall, M., Kupfer, D. J. & Reynolds, C. F. III. (2003). Healthy older adults' sleep predicts all-cause mortality at 4 to 19 years of follow up. *Psychosomatic Medicine*, 65, 63–73.

8. Seifritz, E., MD. (2001). Contribution of sleep physiology to depressive pathophysiology. *Neuropsychopharm.*, 25, 585–588.

9. Roehrs, T. (2000). Sleep physiology and pathophysiology. *Clinical Cornerstone*, 2(5), 1–15.

10. Roth, T., Roehrs, T., Carskadon, M. & Dement, W. C. (1994). Daytime sleepiness and alertness. In M. H. Kryger, T. Roth & W. C. Dement (Eds.). *Principals and practice of sleep medicine*. Philadelphia: W. B. Saunders Co.

11. Doghramji, K. (1989). Sleep disorders: A selective update. *Hospital and Community Psychiatry*, 40(1), 29–40.

12. Hauri, P. J. & Orr, W. C. (1982). *The sleep disorders*. Upjohn Co., Kalamazoo, MI.

13. Kandel, E. R. & Schwartz, J. H. (1981). *Principles of neuroscience*. New York: Elsevier North Holland Inc.

14. Karam-Hage, M., MD. (2004). Treating insomnia in patients with substance use/abuse Disorders. *Psychiatric Times,* February, 55–56.

15. Stahl, S. M. (1999). Awakening to the psychopharmacology of sleep and

   arousal: Novel neurotransmitters and wake-promoting drugs. *J. Clinical Psychiatry*, 63(4), 339–402.

16. Preston, J. D., PsyD, O'Neal, J. H., MD & Talaga, M. C., RPH, MA. (1997). *Handbook of clinical psychopharmacology for therapists* (2ed.). Oakland, CA: New Harbinger.

17. Alternative sleep aids. Retrieved Apr. 9, 2004, from http://www.healingdeva.com/selena2.htmSuggestedSupplements

18. Lin, L., Faraco, J., Li, R., Kadotani, H., Rogers, W., Lin, X., Qui, X. & de Jong, P. J. (1999). The sleep disorder canine narcolepsy is caused by a mutation in the hypocretin (orexin) receptor 2 gene. *Cell*, 98, 365–376.

19. Hungs, M. & Mignot, E. (2001). Hypocretin/orexin, sleep and narcolepsy. *Bioessays*, 23, 397–408.

20. Scammell, T. E., Estabrooke, I. V., McCarthy, M. T., Chemelli, R., Yanagisawa, M., Miller, M. S., & Saper, C. B. (2000). Hypothalamic arousal regions are activated during modafinil-induced wakefulness. *J. Neuroscience*, 20, 8620–8.

21. McClellan, K. J. & Spencer, C. M. (1998). Modafinil: A review of its pharmacology and clinical efficacy in the management of narcolepsy. *CNS Drugs*, 9(4), 311–24.

22. Borgen, L. A., Cook, H. N., Hornfeldt, C. S. & Fuller, D. E. (2002). Sodium Oxybate (GHB) for treatment of cataplexy. *Pharmacotherapy*, 22(6), 798–799.

23. Idzikowski, C. (2000). *Learn to sleep well.* London: Duncan Baird.

24. Bootzin, R. R. & Perlis, M. L. (1992). Nonpharmacological treatments of insomnia. *J. Clinical Psychiatry*, 53, 37–41.

Chapter 2

Treatment of Insomnia & Anxiety Disorders

L ong before anyone ever heard of psychiatrists or psychotherapists, people were using alcohol, laudanum, chloral hydrate, kava, and many other substances to help them sleep and to control anxiety. Since the development of barbiturates in the early 20th century, hundreds of drugs to induce sleep and decrease anxiety have been added to the pharmacopia. The benzodiazepines (BZs) were introduced in the 1970's to avoid some of the adverse effects caused by the barbiturates. More recently, the hypnotic agents zaleplon/Sonata and zolpidem/Ambien, 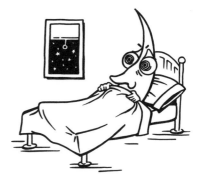 which are in a class of drugs called imidazopyridines, were developed with the hope of avoiding some of the difficulties that occur with the BZs.[1] Today, many psychotherapy clients routinely take a wide variety of substances to decrease their anxiety and to help with their sleep problems; these include prescription drugs, over-the-counter compounds, herbs, and supplements.

Manufacturers continually refine drugs in an attempt to isolate specific effects and to eliminate adverse effects. For example, medical science has long desired a drug that reduces anxiety but does not induce sleep, another that can be used as an anesthetic and not cause a hangover, and still another that prevents seizures and yet would not make patients sleepy. Although researchers are getting closer, as of today no one has been successful in finding compounds that completely achieve these goals.

At normal doses, all sedative-hypnotic drugs act on the *reticular* and *thalamic projection systems* in the brain and are CNS depressants.

Both of these brain centers play an important role in the maintenance of wakefulness. At high doses, some sedative-hypnotic drugs depress the CNS so much that they can induce a coma and cause a fatal *respiratory depression* (sedation of the brain centers that control breathing).

Sedative-Hypnotic Drugs

Effects on sleep architecture

Sedatives (sometimes called "hypnotic" or "sleep-inducing" drugs) decrease the time it takes between lying down to the onset of Stage 1 sleep. Taking sedatives or antianxiety drugs as a sleep aid more frequently than once or twice a week leads to a decrease in REM. After this, when a person stops taking the drug, there will be a period of REM rebound when the time spent in REM is increased. Since REM is a "light" stage of sleep, this results in a greater number of spontaneous awakenings each night. This will be experienced as an increase in sleep disturbance.[2] (See Fig. 2.1.)

As we have seen in Chapter 1, during a normal night of sleep a person progresses from Stage 1 to Delta sleep, then back from Delta sleep to Stage 1, then into the first REM period. This first sleep cycle usually takes from 60 to 120 minutes, with an average of about 90 minutes.[1] (See Fig. 1.1.)

Since REM sleep is very close to the wakeful state, one is easily awakened during REM. The reason that people remember their dreams is believed to be due to the proximity of REM to wakefulness. Throughout the night, periods of Delta sleep typically become shorter and periods of REM get longer. As the time spent asleep progresses, people experience more dreams, and a greater percentage of time is spent in the lighter stages of sleep, which in turn leads to more frequent awakenings towards morning.[1]

Tolerance to sedatives

Tolerance (see Appendix E) to the effects of most sedative drugs develops with regular use.[3] For optimal effect, sedatives must be taken only once or twice a week; to prevent REM rebound, it is essential they not be taken every night. If sedatives are taken intermittently, the patient will have the desired result of fewer awakenings on the nights that the drug is taken. Even with an intermittent dose regimen, Delta sleep, if not eliminated, may be greatly reduced. This reduction can result in feelings of not being rested. The specific medical and/or psychological consequences of diminished sleep are currently being investigated.[4]

The respiratory centers in the CNS do not habituate quickly to these drugs, whereas the neurons responsible for sleep induction do. This habituation (decrease in effect) leads some people to increase their dose to obtain the desired sedative effect. Since the respiratory centers in the CNS do not habituate at the same rate as the sleep and arousal centers, increasing one's dose can lead to a fatal respiratory depression.

BARBITURATES

Many barbiturates with differing properties have been synthesized. Once widely prescribed for anxiety and for sleep problems, quite a few are still in use today, primarily as anesthetic agents during surgery and to treat seizure disorders like epilepsy.

Barbiturates are classified into several categories as determined by their rates of absorption, distribution, metabolism, and excretion. The shorter-acting compounds are often used as intravenous anesthetics, whereas the longer-acting compounds, including phenobarbitol/Luminal, are frequently used for controlling seizure disorders. Some barbiturates have proven useful in the treatment of bipolar disorder, particularly for the manic symptoms, and for controlling the aggressive behavior in patients with explosive disorder. Barbiturates are not the first drugs of choice for treatment of these psychiatric disorders, but are tried if other drugs are not effective, are problematic in some way (e.g., the patient has drug allergies), or if there are other medical contraindications.

Enzymatic and *pharmacodynamic tolerances* (see Appendix E, p. 203) develop with barbiturates. Both types of tolerance contribute to a decrease in effectiveness. Barbiturates, taken orally or dissolved and injected, can be abused to induce euphoria.

BENZODIAZEPINES (BZs)

The BZs were developed with the hope of finding a group of sedative and antianxiety drugs that did not cause physical dependence and had a lower lethality than barbiturates. The attempt was partly successful, in that BZs reduce anxiety, decrease sleep latency, and have a very low risk of lethality if not combined with other sedatives or with alcohol. For people with a history of addiction, time has shown that BZs can also be very addictive .

The BZs are a safer treatment for anxiety than barbiturates because they depress the respiratory centers of the brain less. The BZs block nervous system stimulation that originates in the *reticular formation* of the brain stem. They also diminish neuronal activity in the areas of the brain associated with emotion: the *septal region*, *amygdala*, hypothalamus, and *hippocampus*. The decrease in neuronal activity in these

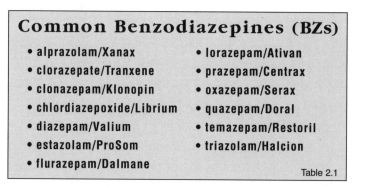

Common Benzodiazepines (BZs)

- alprazolam/Xanax
- clorazepate/Tranxene
- clonazepam/Klonopin
- chlordiazepoxide/Librium
- diazepam/Valium
- estazolam/ProSom
- flurazepam/Dalmane
- lorazepam/Ativan
- prazepam/Centrax
- oxazepam/Serax
- quazepam/Doral
- temazepam/Restoril
- triazolam/Halcion

Table 2.1

IMPORTANT: Patients should always be cautioned never to drink alcohol in combination with BZs or any sedative drug.

areas is most likely responsible for reducing anxiety and emotional reactivity, and also for the memory problems associated with BZ use.

As with all sedatives, BZs interact with alcohol. This interaction leads to an increase in the effect of both drugs. Combining BZs with alcohol greatly increases the likelihood of a fatal respiratory depression.

Use of the BZs in anxiety disorders

The most appropriate long-term use for BZs is in the treatment of Generalized Anxiety Disorder (GAD) and Panic Disorder. GAD is characterized by sustained "free-floating" anxiety, whereas Panic Disorder is characterized by episodes of intense anxiety. Both GAD and Panic Disorder have a genetic component and aggregate in families.[2] Evidence suggests that a defect in the gamma-amino butyric acid (GABA) system is a cause in anxiety disorders.[1]

It is noteworthy that the main site of action of BZs is the *limbic system* of the brain. During a panic attack, the limbic system is sending many excitatory impulses to the cortex. The BZs act to inhibit the limbic system, which reduces the anticipatory anxiety that precipitates a panic attack. Often this reduction is enough to prevent the attack. Patients do not seem to habituate to the anxiety-reducing effect of the BZs.

One disadvantage of taking BZs daily for anxiety is that there will be a rebound in anxiety symptoms if the BZ is discontinued. BZs are particularly useful for anxiety because they can be taken as needed and do not have to be taken on a daily basis.

When taken for anxiety, the effect of BZs on sleep depends on the specific BZ and the time of day it is taken. If a short or medium-acting BZ is taken early in the day it will have little affect on sleep.

Adverse effects & tolerance to BZs

Initial exposure to BZs usually causes some impairment in cognitive functioning, in particular difficulty learning new information (*anterograde amnesia*). If the BZ is taken daily, after about two weeks some tolerance to the cognitive impairment and memory difficulties usually develops. Little tolerance develops to the antianxiety effect or to the impairment of psychomotor performance. This means that even though one may feel mentally clearer, psychomotor skills (e.g., driving) continue to be impaired. Use of BZs provides an example of how tolerance to different effects of a drug develops at varying rates, and how this can have serious consequences.

BZ addiction & hangover

In general, the more quickly a drug is metabolized, the greater its addictive potential. The faster-acting BZs are usually prescribed to help with sleep. In contrast, the slowly-metabolized BZs (the ones usually prescribed for anxiety disorders) tend to accumulate in the body. Accumulation leads to a decrease in alertness and hand-eye coordination, which because of the slower metabolism, may even continue the day after the BZ is taken.

Effects of BZs on sleep

Tolerance to the sleep-inducing effect of BZs develops quickly, causing a loss in effectiveness for the treatment of insomnia after about two weeks of continuous use.[3] For an optimal sleep-inducing effect, BZs should only be taken every three or four days.

There are typical changes in sleep patterns that occur after taking a sedative on a long-term basis (over two weeks of daily use) and a drug-induced insomnia results.[3] After this point, if the sedative is stopped, a period of rebound insomnia will occur and the sleep pattern will be even more disrupted than it was with medication. This rebound effect, and the resulting increase in sleep difficulties, is the reason that it is very difficult for most people to stop taking sleep medication after they have become habituated to it.[1]

The graphs in Fig. 2.1 illustrate the effects of sedatives on sleep architecture:

Effects of Sedatives on
Sleep Architecture

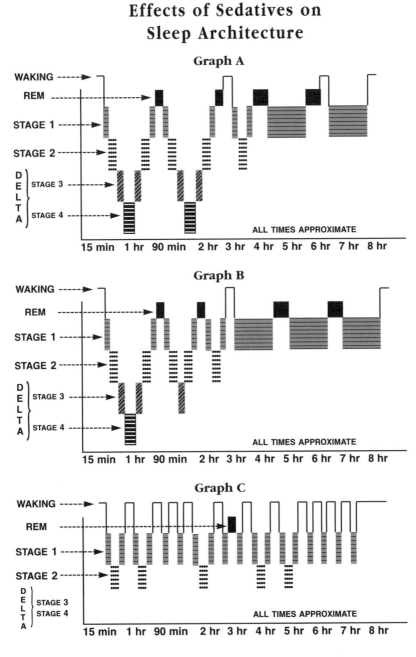

Figure 2.1   (adapted from Kandel & Schwartz 1981)

Graph A: Represents the sleep pattern of someone who woke up twice during the night and was complaining of too many early-morning awakenings. This person wanted medication to help with sleep.

Graph B: Shows the sleep pattern of the same patient just after beginning treatment with a sedative. There are fewer early-morning awakenings, but the periods of deep sleep are already greatly reduced.

Graph C: Represents the patient's sleep patterns after two weeks of taking the sedative on a daily basis. The number of spontaneous awakenings has increased and all periods of deep sleep have been eliminated.[1]

Effects of BZs on memory & pain

BZs interfere with the ability to remember new information by inhibiting nerve transmission in the hippocampus. This interference with memory leads to an interesting capacity that the BZs have with regard to pain. Although BZs have no anesthetic or analgesic effect, they do interfere with the retention of the memory of pain, and are often given along with anesthetic compounds for various medical procedures. This leads patients to think that they had little or no pain, but what in fact was diminished was not the pain itself, but the memory of the pain. When an observer is present for a painful procedure in which a BZ has been given to a patient, the observer will report that the patient reacted as if there was pain, but the patient, if asked later, will have no memory of it. The question is: if one does not remember pain, how much does it matter whether or not it occurred? (A little like the riddle of the tree falling in the forest: if there's no one there to hear it, does it make any sound?) Somatic psychotherapists believe that the memory of the pain is held by the body even if the person cannot remember it.

Most people who take BZs on a daily basis will develop a partial tolerance to the memory-impairment effect in about three weeks. If the BZ is discontinued, memory usually returns to normal after about one week.

Withdrawal from BZs & other sedative-hypnotic drugs

The symptoms of withdrawal from a sedative-hypnotic drug are often the same as the symptoms for which it was originally taken. If the drug has been taken at high dose levels for a long time, withdrawal may lead to more severe symptoms such as confusion, seizures, hallucinations, and delusions.[5]

When longer-acting forms of drugs are used, withdrawal symptoms can appear several days after the last dose, and may continue for two to three weeks. With shorter-acting forms, the symptoms appear sooner, are more intense, but abate more quickly. The exact length of time it will take for any one person to withdraw from any drug depends on many factors, such as dose, metabolic rate, and personality, and cannot be predicted.[5]

Frequent symptoms of withdrawal from BZs

- irritability
- restlessness
- insomnia
- muscle tension

Other possible symptoms of BZ withdrawal

- seizures
- blurred vision
- feelings of weakness
- increased blood pressure
- hypersensitivity to light and sound
- nightmares
- rapid heartbeat
- aches and pains

The psychiatrist needs to oversee a slow tapering of the dose to ease the symptoms of withdrawal. The usual regimen is to reduce the dose 5% to 10% a day for a week or two. When a patient is taking a short-acting drug, a longer-acting preparation may be substituted first, then tapered off. The procedure of switching from a shorter-acting to a longer-acting compound usually prevents seizures and lessens discomfort.[5]

IMPORTANT: The danger of seizures is highest more than one week after the last dose of the sedative.

IMIDAZOPYRIDINES

This class of hypnotic drugs, the imidazopyridines, includes zaleplon/Sonata and zolpidem/Ambien, which are now being used for sleep difficulties. Because they are metabolized rapidly, there is less drowsiness or drug

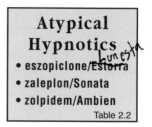

Atypical Hypnotics
- eszopiclone/Estorra ~~Lunesta~~
- zaleplon/Sonata
- zolpidem/Ambien

Table 2.2

hangover the next day. If drugs in this class do prove to be safer than the BZs, and not potentially addictive, they may replace the BZs as a treatment for sleep problems.

Another drug in this class, eszopiclone/Estorra, was approved for use in March, 2004. The manufacturer claims that this drug remains effective when taken consecutively for many weeks.[6]

Other Antianxiety Medications

BUSPIRONE

Buspirone (which is unrelated structurally to the BZs and other sedatives) does not have muscle relaxant, sedative, or anticonvulsant effects. It does not bind to the BZ receptors, although it does bind to 5-HT and DA receptors.[2]

A major advantage of buspirone is that it has a very low risk of lethality if taken by itself. It can be used by people who drink since it does not add to the effects of alcohol or other drugs that depress the CNS. In addition, it does not cause euphoria, so there is a low risk of addiction. This drug does not cause impairment of cognitive functioning, memory, or psychomotor skills.[2]

Buspirone seems to be as effective as the BZs in the treatment of GAD, and has been found effective for treating depressive symptoms in anxious patients. This is a major advantage, since many other drugs used to treat anxiety increase symptoms of depression.[2]

Adverse effects of buspirone

The frequency of adverse effects with buspirone is very low. Some people may experience dizziness, headache, nausea, and diarrhea. These symptoms decrease if the person stays on the drug long enough to become habituated (usually one or two weeks). The major drawback with buspirone is that it is designed to be taken on a daily basis; unlike the BZs, buspirone is not to be taken "as needed."[2]

Other Drugs for Anxiety and Sedation

- buspirone/BuSpar
- clonidine/Catapres
- escitalopram/Lexapro
- diphenhydramine/Benadryl
- gabapentin/Neurontin
- hydroxyzine/Atarax, Vistaril
- melatonin
- paroxetine/Paxil
- propranolol/Inderal
- sodium oxybate/Xyrem

Table 2.3

PROPRANOLOL

The drug propranolol/Inderal was developed for the treatment of high blood pressure and cardiac arrhythmias, for which it is very effective and has few adverse effects. This drug is useful for people with panic attacks because it decreases the *enteroceptive* (internally generated) cues of anxiety, specifically rapid heartbeat and increased blood pressure. In people with a history of panic attacks, often an internal signal of anxiety, such as rapid heartbeat, can precipitate an attack.

Although used for panic attacks, propranolol has not been tested and approved as an antianxiety medication; this is considered an "off label" use. Propranolol should not be used as an antianxiety medication for people with cardiac problems. Serious rebound phenomena can occur if this medication is stopped abruptly. In particular, this can cause an increase in cardiac irregularities that can lead to a potentially fatal disruption in heart functioning.

Propranolol does not interfere with memory or psychomotor performance. Because it decreases stage fright, it has become popular with public speakers, musicians, performers, and people taking licensure examinations. For a person with a history of substance abuse, propranolol may be the most appropriate drug as an ongoing antianxiety medication because it does not produce a "high," and therefore has no potential for abuse.[2]

Adverse effects of propranolol

Some of the possible adverse effects of propranolol are:

- a potentially dangerous worsening of asthma
- nausea • vomiting • gastrointestinal (GI) symptoms

GLUTAMATE RECEPTOR (mGLU) AGONIST

LY354740 is a novel compound that reduces glutamate transmission in brain regions involved in anxiety and stress. In a preclinical study, this drug reduced anxiety without causing a sedative effect. If determined to be safe and effective and approved by the FDA, it offers advantages over antianxiety agents which have sedation as an undesirable side effect.[7]

OVER-THE-COUNTER DRUGS (ANTIHISTAMINES)

Over-the-counter (OTC) sleep aids such as Tylenol PM often contain the antihistamines diphenhydramine/Benadryl or doxylamine. These aid sleep by causing a blockage of histamine receptors. This blockage of histamine neurons induces sleep by shortening sleep latency.[8] These preparations are usually safe, but there is a wide variety of responses to this drug. Some people do not get sleepy, and among those who do, some develop a tolerance to the sleep-induction effect quite rapidly, sometimes after taking the drug only once or twice.[9] Some people who experience improved sleep have a drug hangover the next day. This can usually be prevented by taking the antihistamine earlier in the evening.[8]

Because they are considered relatively safe, antihistamines have been widely used for the treatment of insomnia in children and the elderly (though recent studies indicate that there may be some cognitive impairment in the elderly who use them as a sleep aid).[10] They are sometimes used to treat psychotic symptoms and behavior disorders in children (the decrease in symptoms may be a response to the general CNS sedation). Antihistamine use also leads to a suppression of REM sleep and to a period of REM rebound when the drug is withdrawn.[8] For some people, antihistamines are very effective for sleep problems when used intermittently.

Risk of taking antihistamines during pregnancy

There is some indication that antihistamines may cause birth defects if taken during the first trimester. In general, it is best that no medications be taken during pregnancy.[11]

Direct Relevance to Psychotherapy

Clients frequently come into treatment with sleep problems; many are already taking sleep medications and want to stop. If a client is habituated to a sleep medication, a medical consultation is necessary before withdrawal is attempted.

Sedatives are effective as antiseizure medications because they increase the seizure threshold (i.e., they decrease the likelihood of a seizure by depressing the CNS). Because of this effect, withdrawal from these drugs leads to an increased likelihood of seizures or convulsions; these can be fatal. Other disturbing symptoms frequently experienced during sedative withdrawal are agitation, hallucinations, and disorientation. When sedatives are withdrawn, REM rebound occurs, leading to an increase in the symptoms of insomnia. The worsening of the insomnia may last until the withdrawal period is over, which sometimes takes weeks.

It is not unusual for clients who are taking medication for sleep problems to report that their problems have continued despite the drugs, and that they have increased their dose hoping to obtain the desired effect of a better night's sleep. Unfortunately, most people do not know that increasing the dose will not, in the long run, improve sleep. Using these medications too frequently often results in a dangerous cycle of increasing dosage and continued poor sleep. If a client reports these problems, and wants to continue using a sedative, the psychotherapist should recommend a medication reevaluation by a psychiatrist.

References for Chapter 2

1. Kandel, E. R. & Schwartz, J. H. (1981). *Principles of neuroscience.* NY, NY: Elsevier North Holland Inc.
2. Goa, K. L. & Ward, A. (1986). *Drugs, 32,* 114.
3. Armitage, R., Yonkers, K., Cole, D. & Rush, J. (1997). A multicenter, double-blind comparison of the effects of nefazodone and fluoxetine on sleep architecture and quality of sleep in depressed outpatients. *J. Clinical Psychopharm.,* 17(3), 161–168.
4. Dew, M. A., PhD, Hoch, C. C., Buysse, D. J., Monk, T. H., Begley, A. E., Houck, P. R., Hall, M., Kupfer, D. J. & Reynolds, C. F. III. (2003). Healthy older adults' sleep predicts all-cause mortality at 4 to 19 years of follow up. *Psychosomatic Medicine,* 65, 63–73.
5. Chiang, W. K., MD & Goldfrank, L. R., MD. (1990). Substance withdrawal. *Emergency Medicine Clinics of North America,* 8(3), 613–631.
6. Estorra improves sleep for insomnia patients *FDA News.com.* May 27, 2003. Retrieved Jan. 18 2004, from http://www.fdanews.com/dailies/dpa/1_91/news/13837-1.html
7. Klodzinska, A., Chojnaka-Wojcik, E., Palucha, A., Branski, P., Popik, P. & Plic, A. (1999). Potential anti-anxiety, anti-addictive effects of LY354740, a selective group II glutamate metabotropic receptors agonist in animal models. *Neuropharm.,* 38(12), 1831–1839.
8. Gengo, F., Gabros, C. & Miller, J. K. (1989). The pharmacodynamics of diphenhydramine-induced drowsiness and changes mental performance. *Clin. Pharm. Therapeutics,* 45(1), 15–21.
9. Richardson, G. S., Roehrs, T. A., Rosenthal, L., Koshorek, G. & Roth, T. (2002). Tolerance to daytime sedative effects of H1 antihistamines. *J. Clin. Psychopharm.,* 22(5), 511–515.
10. Simons, F. E., Fraser, T. G., Maher, J., Pillay, N. & Simons, K. J. (1999). Central nervous system effects of H1-receptor antagonists in the elderly. *Ann. Allergy Asthma Immunol.,* 82(2), 157–160.
11. Miller, A. A. (2002). Diphenhydramine toxicity in a newborn: A case report. *J. Perinatol.,* 20(6), 390-391.

Chapter 3
Alcohol: Use & Abuse

A lcohol (also known as ethyl alcohol, ethanol, and grain alcohol) has a molecular structure unlike any other drug discussed in this book. Although the sedative-hypnotic drugs and alcohol are not chemically related, their behavioral, physiological, and psychological effects are very similar.

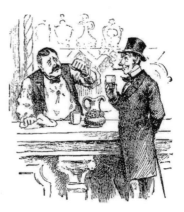

Alcohol, one of the most widely used drugs in western culture, is the intoxicant found in beer, wine, and hard liquor. There is evidence in ancient art and ceramics that alcohol has been used for its intoxicating qualities for at least 6,000 years. Today, between 10.5 million and 14 million Americans suffer from alcoholism, and at least 100,000 deaths each year are associated with alcohol abuse. These fatalities are caused both directly, by damage to the liver and other organs, and indirectly, by automobile or other accidents resulting from alcohol intoxication. Alcohol consumption plays a part in 30%–50% of all traffic fatalities in America.[1] A driver who has had one alcoholic drink is 11 times more likely to be involved in a traffic accident than one who has not had any.

For most people, moderate use (defined as fewer than two drinks per day) is not a health danger (as long as they do not drive afterward). There is some evidence that one or two glasses of red wine per day may even have some health benefits due to the antioxidant properties in the grapes. The main problem with alcohol use is that many people cannot limit their drinking. The risk of abuse and addiction for these individuals is increased by alcohol's ready availability and low cost.

It is clear that there is a genetic component to alcohol addiction. The chance that the siblings and offspring of alcoholics will become alcoholics themselves is seven times greater than for the general population. Males are particularly at risk. The chance of the average man becoming an alcoholic is 3% to 5%, whereas for the son of an alcoholic the estimates range from 20% to 50%. For women, the chances of becoming alcoholic are between 0.1% and 1%, but for the daughters of alcoholics the risk increases to between 3% and 8%.[1] It is important that close relatives of alcoholics are made aware of their greatly increased risk.

The Process of Intoxication

Alcohol is a small molecule that is soluble in both fat and water. The combination of small size and solubility make it easy for the alcohol

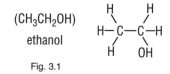

(CH_3CH_2OH)
ethanol

Fig. 3.1

molecule to cross the *blood-brain barrier* (see Appendix B, p. 174). This means that the brain is not protected from high levels of alcohol in the blood stream; the concentration of alcohol present in the CNS is the same as it is in the rest of the body.[2,3]

The initial experience after consuming alcohol is usually a feeling of stimulation. This is a result of a disinhibition in the CNS, which takes place at low doses for all sedative-hypnotic compounds. The first part of the brain to be affected is the cortical area; this causes feelings of euphoria accompanied by a decrease in cognitive and judgmental functions.

Various parts of the brain differ in their sensitivity to alcohol. The part that keeps us awake, the *reticular activating system* (RAS), is highly sensitive to alcohol, while the part that controls respiration, the *medulla oblongata*, is the least sensitive area. This differential sensitivity serves as a life-preserver for heavy drinkers, who will usually pass out due to the general depression of the CNS before the level of intoxication is reached where respiration becomes critically impaired. Impairment of respiration requires at least a 0.4% *blood alcohol concentration* (BAC). Estimating BAC is complicated by many factors, such as weight, age, drug use, liver condition, and food and water consumption. The only way to accurately determine BAC is with a blood test or a breathalyzer test.

Effects of Chronic Alcohol Use

The main long-term effects of alcohol use are changes in the hippocampal area of the brain (which is important in the processes of learning and memory), and liver damage in the form of fat deposits, fibrosis, nodule formations, and cirrhosis, all of which combine to impair normal liver functions. Although there is evidence that some of the damage to the liver and the brain is due to dietary and vitamin deficiencies, alcohol also causes direct damage to the cells of both these vital organs.[4]

Pharmacodynamic & metabolic tolerance

Tolerance to alcohol varies widely among individuals. Chronic ingestion leads to both pharmacodynamic and metabolic tolerances (see Appendix E). Pharmacodynamic tolerance results from prolonged exposure of the CNS to alcohol. This exposure causes the cells of the CNS to become less sensitive to alcohol. When this occurs, a higher BAC is required to attain the desired euphoric effect. Metabolic (enzymatic) tolerance reaches an upper limit and then remains constant. If liver damage occurs, enzymatic tolerance may decrease.

Cross-tolerance

Cross-tolerance can develop between alcohol and other CNS depressants. This means that a person who already has a tolerance to any sedative-hypnotic drug may require a higher dose of alcohol to attain the desired level of intoxication. The cross-tolerance is the result of both pharmacodynamic and metabolic factors. This cross-tolerance does not raise the amount of alcohol that constitutes a lethal dose.

WERNICKE'S DISEASE

Wernicke's disease is seen in chronic alcoholics, and is mainly caused by a deficiency in vitamin B_1 (thiamin).[4] Many alcoholics get their daily caloric intake from alcohol rather than from food, resulting in multiple vitamin deficiencies. This disease will not occur if B-vitamin supplements are taken, even if drinking continues. The onset of Wernicke's disease is usually sudden. Symptoms include:

- disorientation
- apathy
- ataxia (dizziness)
- delirium
- drowsiness
- nystagmus (uncontrollable horizontal eye movements)[4]

Immediate treatment with B vitamins, administered either intramuscularly (i.m.) or, for the most rapid effect, intravenously (i.v.), may reduce permanent damage to the CNS. Treatment consists of continued daily administration of oral B vitamins.[4]

KORSAKOFF'S PSYCHOSIS

Korsakoff's psychosis is characterized by a severe disturbance in recent memory. It is found in 80% of patients who have been diagnosed with Wernicke's disease. Korsakoff's may begin insidiously, with no overt symptoms, or it may appear suddenly following a series of *delirium tremens* (DTs). The patient has anterograde amnesia for all events that occur after the onset of the illness, and often for events that occurred in the weeks or months before the onset, as well as *retrograde amnesia* (inability to recall already-learned facts). The patient is unaware of having amnesia, and uses *confabulation* (making things up) to cover up the memory deficits. The anterograde amnesia disorients the sufferer as to time, and although cognitive functioning remains stable, the patient is unable to learn even very simple new information like remembering the time of day. The person remains alert, is generally cheerful, and seems unaware of the disability.

Prognosis for these patients is poor because there is usually a continuance of alcohol consumption.[4]

Autopsies performed on people with Korsakoff's psychosis show damage to the cells of the hippocampus, parts of the hypothalamus, and the thalamus. The damage is permanent, and is thought to be the result of the B-vitamin deficiency.[4]

FETAL ALCOHOL SYNDROME (FAS)

FAS is a disease of the newborn that occurs when alcohol is consumed during pregnancy. Obvious symptoms of FAS may occur with as few as two drinks per day, and there is evidence of subtle damage to the CNS at even lower levels. The syndrome is seen in the babies of 4 out of 100 heavy-drinking mothers, and is the third-leading cause of birth defects associated with mental retardation.[4] The severity of the symptoms is proportional to the amount of alcohol consumed. FAS defects include:

- low birth weight • cardiovascular defects
- joint and limb abnormalities
- abnormalities in facial structure
- mental retardation (can be quite severe)
- microcephaly (infant's brain is underdeveloped)[5]

WARNING: No completely safe level of alcohol use during pregnancy has been determined.[5]

Withdrawal from Alcohol

Withdrawal symptoms usually begin 24 to 48 hours after the last drink (although they may not appear for up to three weeks and can even begin during a period of high alcohol intake).[2] Many in-patient programs use BZs or anticonvulsants to ease the symptoms of alcohol withdrawal and to decrease the risk of seizures. When BZs are used, the patient is first taken off the alcohol and then slowly tapered off the BZ. Frequently seen mild symptoms of alcohol withdrawal include:

- shaking
- sweating
- anxiety
- anorexia
- vomiting
- abdominal cramps

In more serious cases of withdrawal, auditory and visual hallucinations and paranoid delusions are sometimes present.[6]

DELIRIUM TREMENS (DTs)

The severe alcohol withdrawal syndrome is known as delirium tremens (DTs). The mortality rate is between 4% and 15%. DTs begin with anxiety attacks, confusion, poor sleep, marked sweating, and profound depression. Increases in pulse rate, sweating, and body temperature parallel the progress of the delirium. The acute period generally lasts from two to ten days, but is sometimes more prolonged. Usually the symptoms of DTs begin to abate within 12 to 24 hours.[4]

Epilepsy & alcohol withdrawal

When chronic alcohol use is stopped, the CNS becomes hyperexcitable; this increases the risk of seizures. Although the period of hyperexcitability can last for several days, the seizure risk peaks within 8 to 10 hours after the last dose of alcohol. CNS hyperexcitability is particularly dangerous for epileptics, who are already at an increased risk for seizures. Epileptics who have become addicted to alcohol must be monitored very closely during withdrawal. *Grand mal* seizures may develop within 48 hours after the last drink.[6]

A study by Reoux demonstrated that divalproax sodium/Depakote, a drug used to control seizures, can lessen symptoms during alcohol withdrawal. Use of divalproax sodium would eliminate the need to use BZs for people who have moderately severe symptoms of alcohol withdrawal. Clinical evaluations for this use of divalproax sodium are under way.[7]

> **WARNING: The withdrawal process from alcohol can be fatal even under medical supervision.**[6]

Pharmacological Aids for Abstinence

Disulfiram

The drug disulfiram/Antabuse is sometimes prescribed as a deterrent to alcohol consumption. Taking disulfiram and then drinking alcohol will have unpleasant and possibly even fatal consequences. Disulfiram interacts with anything that contains alcohol and with many medications. Any exposure to alcohol, even in small amounts, may cause symptoms of illness. There can be a risk to health if disulfiram is taken when other medical conditions are present.[4] (See Fig. D1, p. 192, for the action of disulfiram on alcohol metabolism.)

The theory behind the use of disulfiram is that a patient's fear of experiencing the unpleasant effects that result from combining disulfiram and alcohol will discourage drinking. In general, taking disulfiram without some form of psychotherapy is not effective. Some people drink while taking disulfiram and become ill, others stop taking disulfiram rather than stop drinking. The lack of success of disulfiram in decreasing alcoholism illustrates that punishment is not the optimal method for changing behavior.[8]

Naltrexone for alcoholism

Studies show promising results using the opioid *antagonist* naltrexone/Trexan/ReVia in the treatment of alcoholism.[9, 10] (See Appendix D for an explanation of the concepts of *agonist* and antagonist). Naltrexone was originally developed to treat the craving experienced by diacetylmorphine (heroin) addicts during withdrawal (see pps. 90, 119–120). It binds to CNS opioid receptors without producing any sense of euphoria. By preventing the alcohol molecule from binding to the opioid receptors, rewarding effects are diminished, and craving for alcohol are decreased. This makes it easier for someone who has relapsed into drinking to return to abstinence. Behavioral therapy alone reduces relapses to 50%. The combination of behavioral therapy and naltrexone therapy reduces relapses to 20%.[8]

Calcium acetylhomotaurinate

Calcium acetylhomotaurinate/Acamprosate/Campral is currently under expedited review by the FDA for the treatment of alcoholism (it is not yet approved). Its chemical structure is similar to the amino acids taurine and GABA. It stimulates the inhibitory actions of GABA while acting as an antagonist against the excitatory effects of glutamate. This combination seems to ease the discomfort of abstinence.[8] Studies indicate that twice as many people remain abstinent from alcohol while taking calcium acetylhomotaurinate as those not taking any drug.[9, 11]

Ondansetron

Ondansetron/Zofran is an injectable compound that was originally developed as an antinausea drug for use after surgery or for patients on chemotherapy. It is a 5-HT receptor antagonist that has been shown to halt cravings in early-onset alcoholics.[12]

Topiramate

The antiseizure drug topiramate/Topamax was found to be effective in reducing cravings and signs of anxiety in alcohol-dependent individuals (using the definition for dependence found in the *Diagnostic and Statistical Manual IV*).[13] The researchers believe the drug inhibits the release of DA, and through this mechanism decreases cravings. Subjects reported that the taste of alcohol was changed while taking the drug.[14]

Direct Relevance to Psychotherapy

For a variety of therapeutic and practical reasons, it is not advisable for the psychotherapist to attempt to assess the client's level of alcohol dependency. If a client wants to stop drinking, the safest way to proceed is to recommend that withdrawal be done under medical supervision. No one can predict the severity of the withdrawal reaction for any individual. There may also be medical conditions present which could complicate and increase the dangers during the withdrawal process. The best and safest way to support your client during withdrawal is to recommend a consultation with a psychiatrist or a family-practice physician who will supervise the process and provide whatever medical backup may be needed.

Most therapists believe that alcohol addiction is best treated using a combination of individual psychotherapy and group support. The experience of a group of peers already in recovery provides patients with a new and non-drinking supportive environment. When a person stops drinking, there is great benefit in attending a peer-support group like the 12-Step program developed by Alcoholics Anonymous.[15] As always, the best course of treatment must be determined on an individual basis. In some cases, treatment needs to be more behavioral, while in other cases, long-term psychodynamic therapy may be most appropriate. Regardless of additional methods, continuing in individual psychotherapy is highly recommended,[8] particularly during the early stages of recovery.[16] After the initial phase of breaking through the patient's denial, continued confrontation may not be the most effective means of therapy since it may alienate the client and undermine the therapeutic alliance.

It is essential that the client maintain a constant base of support for sobriety while developing new habits and behaviors as a sober person. Depending on the individual, the process of recovery can, and often does, take many years.

References for Chapter 3

1. National Institute on Alcohol Abuse & Alcoholism/Databases. (2002). Retrieved from www.niaaa.nih.gov/databases.
2. Bonner, A. B. (1994). Biological mechanisms of alcohol dependence. *Current Opinion in Psychiatry*, 7, 262–268.
3. Tabakoff, B. & Hoffman, P. L. (1993). The neurochemistry of Alcohol. *Current Opinion in Psychiatry*, 6, 388–394.
4. *The Merck manual of diagnosis and therapy.* (2001). 17th ed. Rahway, NJ: Merck Sharp & Dohme Research Laboratories.
5. Waterson, E. J. & Murray-Lyon, I. M. (1990). Preventing alcohol-related birth damage: A review. *Social Science and Medicine,* 30, 349–364.
6. Chiang, W. K., MD & Goldfrank, L. R., MD. (1990). Substance withdrawal. *Emergency Medicine Clinics of North America,* 8(3), 613–631.
7. Reoux J. P., Saxon, A. J., Malte, C. A., Sloan, K. & Baer, J. (2001). Divalproax sodium alcohol withdrawal: A randomized double-blind placebo controlled clinical trial. *Alcoho. Clin. Exp. Res.,* 25, 1324–1329.
8. Carpenter, S. (2001). Mixing medication and psychosocial therapy for alcoholism. *Monitor on Psychology*, June, 36–37.
9. Schuckit, M. A. (1997). Science, medicine, and the future: Substance use disorders. *BMJ*, 314, 1605–1608.
10. Krystal, J. H., Cramer, J. A. & Kroll, W. F. (2001). Naltrexone in the treatment of alcohol dependence. *New Eng. J. of Medicine*, 345(24), 1734–1739.
11. Tempesta, E., Janiri, L. & Bignamini, A. (2000). Acamprosate and relapse prevention in the treatment of alcohol dependence: A placebo controlled study. *Alcohol Alcoholism*, 35(2), 202–229.
12. Johnson, B. A. (2000). Ondansetron for reduction of drinking among biologically predisposed alcoholic patients. *JAMA*, 284(8), 36.
13. American Psychiatric Association. (1994). *Diagnostic and statistical manual of mental disorders* (4th ed.). Wash., DC: American Psychiatric Association.
14. Johnson, B. A., Ait-Daoud, N., Bowsen, C. L., Di Clemente, C. C., Roache, J. D. & Lawson, K. (2003). Oral topiramate for treatment of alcohol dependence: A randomized controlled trial. *Lancet*, 361, 1677–85.
15. Alcoholics Anonymous, retrieved Sept. 19, 2003, from http://www.alcoholics-anonymous.org/
16. De Angelis, T. (2001). Today's tried-and-true treatments. *Monitor on Psychology,* June, 48–50.

Chapter 4

Treatment of Depressive Disorders

For those who have dwelt in depression's dark wood and known its inexplicable agony, their return from the abyss is not unlike the ascent of the poet, trudging upward and upward out of hell's black depths and at last emerging into what he saw as the "shining world."

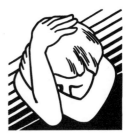

William Styron

The word "depression" is used in psychology to express a complex phenomenon that has a wide variety of both causes and symptoms. There are instances when psychotherapy alone can lead to alleviation of symptoms, while at other times the use of antidepressant medication may be both appropriate and necessary to supplement the psychotherapy.

Two common reasons for considering the use of medication as part of the treatment of depression are to facilitate the psychotherapeutic process and to prevent a potential suicide. Recent studies have found that recurrent depression has a neurodegenerative component. The structure and function of brain cells in depressed patients are disrupted and nerve-cell connections are destroyed, eventually leading to a decline in cognitive functioning.[1] It has been shown that the rate of recovery decreases when depression becomes chronic.[2]

Regardless of the specific cause and type of depression, a commonality in the symptoms and syndromes suggests that the hypothalamus is involved. This is the part of the brain responsible for many of the body's regulatory processes, such as sexual desire, appetite, the ability to sleep, and the ability to experience pleasure.

Many of these processes are altered during depression.

If left untreated with either psychotherapy and/or medication, a first episode of depression can last from four to twelve months, the average length being five months. Some typical symptoms are: a pervasive *dysphoric* (unpleasant) mood, a generalized loss of energy and interests, and a state often described by clients as a loss of the ability to experience pleasure (*anhedonia*).[3]

Evidence for a genetic predisposition

Several factors influence one's chances of developing depression. Studies of twins lend strong support to a genetic component. In monozygotic (identical) twins reared together, the concordance rate for depression is 69%, while for fraternal twins the rate is 13%. The concordance rate of identical twins reared apart is 40% to 60%. Since the concordance rate is not 100%, the presence of factors other than genetics must also influence the development of depression.[4]

Assessment & Symptoms of Depression

Both the symptoms and the etiology of each client's depression must be considered to determine the most appropriate treatment. Even though the symptoms by themselves tell us little about the cause of a patient's depression, the type of symptoms can help the psychotherapist make more effective interventions. A *DSM-IV* diagnosis of depression requires the presence of the following symptoms:

- loss of energy
- decreased sex drive
- difficulty concentrating
- diminished/increased appetite
- guilty, pessimistic, and suicidal thoughts
- disturbed sleep (usually insomnia with early
    morning awakening)
- psychomotor agitation or psychomotor retardation[3]

Other common symptoms are a slowing of PSNS functions, including constipation and decreased salivation. Symptoms are usually worse in the morning, and many people report that towards evening they feel "almost normal." More than 11 million people in the U.S. alone (about four percent of the population) are affected by depression.[5]

Vegetative symptoms: Certain symptoms strongly suggest a biological component or etiology. These vegetative symptoms typically are:
- weight loss or gain
- unreactive mood
- early morning awakening or hypersomnia (sleeping many hours)[3]
- anhedonia
- constipation

Cognitive symptoms: Some symptoms indicate negative thought patterns:
- feelings of helplessness
- difficulty concentrating
- feelings of guilt
- decreased self-esteem[3]

Behavioral symptoms: Another cluster of symptoms reflect a change in normal behavior patterns such as:
- psychomotor retardation (pronounced slowness or lack of movement)
- psychomotor agitation (jittery and increased movement)[3]

As a group, patients with vegetative symptoms are the most likely to need medication for optimal improvement. A person with cognitive symptoms might benefit more from cognitive interventions, or if there are many behavioral symptoms, behavioral interventions might be most effective.

If not properly diagnosed and treated, depression can have serious, long-term consequences. Personal relationships and employment can suffer greatly due to lack of motivation and lack of enjoyment in life. A first episode of depression, if untreated, can persist for as long as a year. Suffering for many months before getting treatment increases the risk of a negative outcome.[1,2,6]

The majority of suicides occur in people who are depressed. There is evidence that patients who are suicidal are frequently under-treated pharmacologically. In one study, only 15% of suicidal patients who had previous suicide attempts, and were hospitalized for depression, were on medication. Only 18% to 20% of these patients had been on medication during the three months prior to their hospitalization. These percentages demonstrate that medication may be under-utilized, even in extreme circumstances.[6]

Subtypes of Depression

It can be useful to classify depression into subtypes according to response to various psychoactive medications. These categories do not correspond directly to *DSM-IV* diagnostic categories because patients are grouped primarily by response to medication.

PSYCHOTIC OR DELUSIONAL DEPRESSION

In a psychotic or delusional depression there is a preponderance of vegetative symptoms with the addition of delusions. The delusions are mood-congruent and usually paranoid in nature. Decreased REM latency is often present. This type of depression responds best to antipsychotic medication. After psychotic symptoms clear, the patient needs to be reevaluated for appropriate interventions.

RECURRENT UNIPOLAR DEPRESSION

This is the most common type of depression.[7] It is generally believed to be due to a biochemical imbalance, and is the type which is most responsive to pharmacological treatment. The first drug of choice is one of the SSRIs. These patients generally have a stable lifestyle, do not have a family history of alcoholism, and do not show signs of a personality disorder. They usually say that they do not know why they are depressed; there is no clear precipitating incident. Recovery rates for this group are good; about 75% improve on SSRIs or *heterocyclic antidepressants* (HCAs), and 70% or more respond to *electroconvulsive therapy* (ECT). These patients have the highest risk of relapse.[2, 8, 9]

DEPRESSIVE SPECTRUM DISORDER

These patients usually present with a chaotic life style which is punctuated by disruptions such as divorce, violence, sexual problems, difficulties with employment, and a family history of alcoholism. Disturbances in eating and sleeping are also frequent. Statistically, they have fewer previous episodes of depression than the unipolar group, and they are somewhat less responsive to SSRIs and HCAs. About 50% are helped by medication.

ATYPICAL DEPRESSION

There are two types of atypical depression: the vegetative type, with symptoms of *hypersomnia* (oversleeping) and *hyperphagia* (compulsive overeating), and the anxiety type, with symptoms of anxiety, restlessness, and nervousness. Panic attacks and phobias may also be present in the anxiety type.

People in this group retain emotional reactivity and do not display the flatness of affect usually seen with depression. They are often hypersensitive to criticism, hyperreactive to rejection, and frequently have gastrointestinal (GI) symptoms. People in this group may respond preferentially to *monoamine oxidase inhibitors* (MAOIs). In current practice, an SSRI is usually tried first so that patients do not have to modify their eating habits (as is necessitated with MAOIs). If the depression is not treated effectively, these patients may eventually become more like unipolar patients.[10]

Note: There is no correlation between "atypical" depression and the use of "atypical" antidepressant drugs.

BIPOLAR DISORDER (see Chapter 5 for a detailed discussion)

This is usually considered to be primarily a biological disorder. Professional opinions differ as to whether the first treatment of choice should be lithium or divalproax sodium. If either of these alone is not effective, antidepressants or thyroid hormone may be added to the patient's regimen to boost response and prevent depression.

Antidepressant Medications by Type

In general, the different types of antidepressant medications are equally effective. The choice of appropriate medication is usually made based upon adverse-effect profiles, prior history of good results, and safety. The initial effect may be one of calming; the patient may begin to feel better before the full effect of the antidepressant medication has been attained. After approximately eight weeks of treatment, all the antidepressant medications will be effective for decreasing a moderately-severe depression in about two-thirds of patients.[6] It may take eight to twelve weeks before antidepressant medications attain their maximum effect.

SELECTIVE SEROTONIN REUPTAKE INHIBITORS (SSRIs)

SSRIs facilitate improvement in mood, decrease hyperreactivity and hypersensitivity, and help to relieve disruptions in sleeping and eating. Prior to the development of the SSRIs, the major difficulty in treating depression with medication was the dangerous combination of the high risk of suicide in this group of patients coupled with the lethality of the available drugs (TCAs and HCAs, see below).[11]

Because of their low level of lethality, SSRIs have made pharmacological intervention much less risky, which has led to the extensive use of this group of drugs for mild to moderate depression. As of March 2000, over 21 million people worldwide were taking just one type of SSRI (Prozac), with millions more taking others. This widespread use of SSRIs contributes to the growing need for psychotherapists to understand the use and misuse of these medications. It is common for every therapy practice to have at least one client on some type of antidepressant medication, usually an SSRI.

Adverse effects of SSRIs

When starting SSRIs many people may experience:

- restlessness
- hyperactive reflexes
- disturbances in sleep patterns and dreams
- irritability
- GI disturbances
- decrease in sexual desire and the ability to achieve orgasm

After a one or two week period of adjustment, many of the initial adverse effects abate.[11]

The FDA issued a health advisory in March, 2004, urging close monitoring of adults and children taking antidepressants and asked manufacturers to include stronger warnings on the labels. Many of the drugs discussed in this book have not been tested as to their specific effects in children, in the geriatric population, or in pregnant women.

Common SSRIs

- citalopram/Celexa
- clomipramine/Anafranil
- escitalopram/Lexapro
- fluvoxamine/Luvox
- fluoxetine/Prozac
- paroxetine/Paxil
- sertraline/Zoloft
- venlafaxine/Effexor
  (an SNRI at higher doses)

Table 4.1

Sexual dysfunction

It is estimated that between 30% and 70% of patients on SSRIs experience some degree of sexual dysfunction.[12] The disturbance in sexual function seems to be the adverse effect most resistant to habituation, and the one that causes the most people to decide to discontinue treatment with SSRIs. Sexual response returns to normal when the SSRI is discontinued. Recent studies show that sildenafil/Viagra may be effective for both men and women as a treatment for the sexual dysfunction caused by SSRI use.[12, 13] Manufacturers claim the newer SSRIs (citalopram/Celexa, venlafaxine/Effexor and escitalopram/Lexapro) have fewer adverse effects, particularly with regard to sexual dysfunction.

Movement disorders

Evidence suggests that SSRIs can cause movement disorders similar to those seen in the *extrapyramidal syndrome* (EPS) caused by antipsychotic medications.[14] (See Chapter 7.)

Toxic serotonin syndrome (TSS)

Toxic serotonin syndrome is a potentially life-threatening complication caused by some *psychotropic* drugs. This syndrome can result from the use of drugs that enhance serotonin activity in the CNS. TSS may be hard to recognize because of the varied and nonspecific nature of its clinical features. Symptoms of TSS are alterations in:

- behavior (agitation, restlessness)
- cognition (disorientation, confusion)
- neuromuscular activity (cramping, hyperactive reflexes, muscle spasms)
- autonomic nervous system function (fever, shivering, sweating, diarrhea) [15]

It is important that the therapist and the client are both aware of these symptoms, particularly if the client is taking more than one serotonin-enhancing drug. If these symptoms occur, immediate referral to a physician is essential so that a medical evaluation and any necessary treatment can begin immediately. TSS can be fatal if not treated promptly.[15]

SEROTONIN/NOREPINEPHRINE REUPTAKE INHIBITORS (SNRIs)

In higher doses, one of the SSRIs, venlafaxine/Effexor, has been shown to also inhibit reuptake of NE.[16] This selectivity is a valuable characteristic because some people respond better to antidepressants that primarily affect the NE system, while others respond better to those that primarily affect the 5-HT system. SNRIs are being

Common SNRIs
- duloxetine/Cymbalta
- venlafaxine/Effexor

Table 4.2

called "dual action" antidepressants because they affect both NE and 5-HT systems. The NE response for venlafaxine is dose-dependent, with NE more affected by higher doses.[16] Patients who do not respond to other SSRIs may respond to venlafaxine, obtaining the benefits of action on NE and 5-HT while taking a medication without the dangers inherent in the tricyclic and heterocyclic antidepressants (discussed below). Another SNRI, duloxetine/Cymbalta, is awaiting FDA approval. This drug exerts NE and 5-HT reuptake inhibition throughout the dose range.

TRICYCLIC & HETEROCYCLIC ANTIDEPRESSANTS (TCAs & HCAs)

Before the advent of the SSRIs, the first choice of medication for depression was either a TCA or an HCA. HCAs were developed to improve on efficacy and decrease the adverse effects seen with TCAs. While no longer the drugs of first choice, both are still used, either for patients already on them who are having successful results with minimal adverse effects, or for patients who do not have an adequate response to SSRIs. There is evidence that more severe depressions may respond preferentially to HCAs rather than to SSRIs.[17] Since TCAs and HCAs have been on the market for many years, an extensive body of research exists as to their efficacy. Twenty-five percent of patients with mild to moderate depression experience remission of symptoms without medication or psychotherapy; the rate of remission is 40% with a placebo, and 70% with TCAs or HCAs.

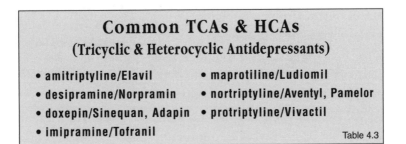

Common TCAs & HCAs
(Tricyclic & Heterocyclic Antidepressants)

- amitriptyline/Elavil
- desipramine/Norpramin
- doxepin/Sinequan, Adapin
- imipramine/Tofranil
- maprotiline/Ludiomil
- nortriptyline/Aventyl, Pamelor
- protriptyline/Vivactil

Table 4.3

Adverse effects of TCAs & HCAs

Some adverse effects are common when starting on TCAs or HCAs. Most frequently seen are:

- initial sedation
- dry mouth
- constipation
- psychomotor slowing
- difficulty concentrating
- muscle twitching
- possible lowering of the seizure threshold
- increased risk of a manic episode (can mean the dose is too high or the diagnosis is bipolar disorder)

Lethality of TCAs & HCAs

This group of medications can be cardiotoxic, particularly for patients with heart disease. In high doses, they can cause a disruption in electrical conduction of the heart.[18] One week's worth of medication, if taken all at once, can be fatal.

It is very dangerous to give patients at greatest risk for suicide a drug that can easily be used for this. Before the availability of the SSRIs, the risk of providing a patient with the means to commit suicide was the major concern for psychiatrists prescribing antidepressant medication. If TCAs or HCAs are being used, and the risk of suicide is high, instituting precautionary measures, such as putting a family member in charge of dispensing medication, or having the person hospitalized so medication is dispensed by staff, is essential.

MONOAMINE OXIDASE INHIBITORS (MAOIs)

The first monoamine oxidase inhibitor (MAOI) found to be effective as an antidepressant was Ipronazid, a drug that was being tested for the treatment of tuberculosis. During clinical trials, some patients who were depressed

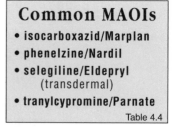

Common MAOIs
- isocarboxazid/Marplan
- phenelzine/Nardil
- selegiline/Eldepryl
  (transdermal)
- tranylcypromine/Parnate

Table 4.4

reported an unexpected elevation in mood. Ipronazid was then tested on patients diagnosed with depression and found to be effective in alleviating their symptoms.

MAOIs work by irreversibly binding to the MAO enzyme and preventing the breakdown of the monoamines NE and 5-HT. The net result of this process is an increase in monoamines in the neuron. The presence of very large amounts of NE can lead to a *hypertensive crisis* (a dangerous elevation of blood pressure). For this reason, if MAOIs are to be used safely, diet must be severely restricted to prevent a hypertensive crisis. This is problematic, since it is very difficult for most people to change their eating habits. Although atypical depression responds preferentially to MAOIs, these drugs are not frequently prescribed due to their strict dietary requirements. Usually, MAOIs are tried when a patient does not respond to SSRIs, SNRIs, or TCAs. Low oral doses of selegiline (an MAO) may be effective as an antidepressant and not require dietary restrictions. (See transdermal selegiline, p. 54.)

Dietary restrictions with MAOIs

Tyramine, an amino acid, is a precursor for NE. Consuming foods that contain large amounts of tyramine leads to an increase in the synthesis of NE, hence the need for a restricted diet. Some food additives also increase the synthesis of NE. A text on nutrition can be consulted for a complete list of the tyramine content of various foods. Some examples of these foods and additives are:

- cyclamates
- overripe avocados
- monosodium glutamate (MSG)
- preserved meats (e.g., salami, bologna)
- pickled foods (e.g., herrings, sauerkraut)
- fermented cheeses (e.g., Blue, Gorgonzola)
- fermented beverages (some beers and wines)
- fermented bean curd products (e.g., soy sauce)

Duration of action

The MAOIs currently available inactivate all MAO present in the nerve cell. This means that no MAO is available in the CNS until more is synthesized. Antidepressant effects are seen for a week or more after the drug is discontinued, or until the nerve cells synthesize adequate amounts of new MAO.

Adverse effects of MAOIs

The most serious risk is the possibility of a hypertensive crisis (see above). A severe headache may signal the onset of a crisis. Other frequent symptoms are:

- increased blood pressure
- *tachycardia* (rapid heartbeat)
- increased body temperature

IMPORTANT: If these symptoms occur, immediate medical attention is required!

These symptoms can indicate a *cardiovascular accident* (stroke or heart attack) which can be fatal. The risk is increased if MAOIs are taken concurrently with common medications such as:

- any TCA or HCA
- amphetamines or other stimulant drugs
- dextromethorphan (in many cough medicines)
- L-dopa (often prescribed for Parkinson's disease)
- over-the-counter and prescription cold preparations
- many other medications

Ingesting significant quantities of any or all of these can cause a hypertensive crisis due to increased levels of NE. The usual treatment consists of administering a particular group of antipsychotic drugs (phenothiazines) which block the action of NE.

Other serious adverse effects can occur if MAOIs are combined with other drugs including:

- phenothiazine tranquilizers
- alcohol
- antihistamines
- barbiturates
- narcotics
- insulin

The combination of the drugs listed above and MAOIs can lead to severe *hypotension* (a serious decrease in blood pressure) that also can be fatal.

MAOIs are contraindicated in the presence of liver or kidney disease, cardiovascular disease, asthma, hypertension, and other diseases. Before prescribing MAOIs, the psychiatrist needs to carefully evaluate each patient to be sure that no contraindications are present.

Discontinuance of MAOIs

As with other antidepressant medications, after a period of being asymptomatic for six to nine months (after a first episode of depression) the patient, in consultation with the psychiatrist and psychotherapist, may decide to discontinue medication. It is important that the dose is tapered slowly and the process closely monitored by a psychiatrist. The patient must be cautioned not to stop taking MAOIs without medical supervision. If MAOIs are withdrawn too quickly, serious conditions can occur (e.g., delirium, delusions, hallucinations, and on occasion, catatonic states).

Due to all the difficulties mentioned above, the MAOIs are rarely prescribed. If a patient is taking an MAOI, it is usually because he or she has been on it for many years and the psychiatrist is reluctant to change a medication if it is working.

Transdermal MAOI

Recent research using transdermal (skin patch) selegiline (an MAOI) shows effectiveness without the serious adverse effects of oral MAOIs. None of the dietary restrictions associated with the oral formulations are necessary using the selegiline patch. Improvement in depressive symptoms was seen in six weeks. Patients also reported improvement in sexual functioning. The only adverse effect seen was a skin rash at the site of the patch. If found to be safe in this form, MAOIs may prove to be very useful for the treatment of depression.[19]

ATYPICAL ANTIDEPRESSANTS & OTHER TREATMENTS

Below are some antidepressant medications that do not fit neatly into the categories already discussed.

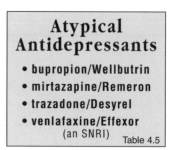

Atypical Antidepressants

- bupropion/Wellbutrin
- mirtazapine/Remeron
- trazadone/Desyrel
- venlafaxine/Effexor
  (an SNRI)

Table 4.5

Bupropion

The drug bupropion/Wellbutrin has been found to be useful as an antidepressant medication when used either alone or in combination with SSRIs. Use of bupropion may improve some aspects of sexual dysfunction associated with SSRIs. Patients taking the combination of bupropion and SSRIs reported an increased desire to engage in sexual activity as well as an increased frequency of sexual activity compared to placebo.[20]

Mirtazapine

The drug mirtazapine/Remeron is one of a group of drugs called 5-HT_2 serotonin receptor antagonists. Since it is sedating, mirtazapine is frequently used to treat depressions when sleep disorders and anxiety symptoms are present. There is some evidence that the onset of improvement with mirtazapine is more rapid than with the SSRIs.[17]

Olanzapine

An antipsychotic medication rather than an antidepressant, olanzapine/Zyprexa has been shown to be effective as an adjunctive agent for depression.[21]

Substance P antagonists (SPAs)

Substance P (SP) antagonists are a new class of compounds being investigated to treat depression and the anxiety sometimes associated with it. Substance P belongs to the neurokinin (NK) family of peptides, and interacts with the NK receptor. It regulates both affective behavior and the perception of pain. It is released in response to stressful stimuli. Studies show that inhibiting the SP-NK receptor system reduces anxiety. Giving subjects SP led to an increase in depressive symptoms and a worsening of mood. Therefore, SPAs may be useful in the treatment of depression. [22]

Neuromodulators used to treat depression

Some of the small peptide molecules that exist normally in our bodies are considered neuromodulators. Many hormones fall into this category. The presence and levels of these substances in the nerve cell and the synapse affect behavior by influencing the neuron's response to neurotransmitters.

Thyroid hormone is one example of a neuromodulator. It is well known that the level of thyroid hormone affects mood. *Hypothyroidism* (too little thyroid hormone) is associated with depressed mood, and *hyperthyroidism* (too much thyroid hormone) is associated with manic states. If the patient's response to antidepressant medication alone is not optimal, psychiatrists may supplement antidepressants with thyroid hormone to enhance the drug's effect(s). Other substances known to affect mood which may function as neuromodulators are the *endorphins* (endogenous opiate-like substances) and the *corticosteroids*.

Electroconvulsive therapy (ECT)

Use of therapeutic shock to treat mental disorders began centuries ago when hot-cold water immersion therapy was tried. In the last century, chemical and electrical methods were developed in the forms of insulin shock and ECT. Insulin shock was discontinued because it was found to be difficult to control, whereas ECT has continued to be refined and is still in use.[8, 9]

ECT is the application of an electrical current, usually to one side of the brain, to induce a CNS seizure. ECT is tried when depression is severe or life-threatening, when there are serious contraindications to antidepressant medications, or when medications have already been tried and have not produced improvement. ECT is also used for treating some psychotic and schizoaffective disorders after medication has been tried and not been effective. Advantages of ECT include:

- no medication side effects
- no risk of suicide due to an overdose
- no interactions with other medications
- no continuous dosing of medication[8, 9]

ECT has a negative reputation and is not used as a first-line treatment (although people who have been treated successfully with ECT often request it if they have a relapse). Some patients and health professionals are adamantly opposed to ECT and consider it inhumane. The most frequent adverse effect is the memory-loss that some patients experience after treatment. Some types of memory-loss are difficult to measure with objective tests, and opinions differ as to the seriousness and extent of this effect, and how much of the loss is caused by ECT. Impairment of memory after ECT is more severe in the elderly.[8, 9]

ECT treatment regimen

The ECT treatment regimen usually consists of a series of four to twelve sessions over a period of two to four weeks. ECT is believed to work by inducing a general CNS seizure; no motor seizure symptoms occur because drugs are used to suppress motor activity. After the seizure, there is a massive alteration in availability of transmitter substances. Specifically, there is an increase in 5-HT levels, and in MAO activity, an increase in the level of DA, and a decrease in the level of NE. ECT may also cause an increase in sensitivity of post-synaptic receptors to all neurotransmitters present. Because there are so many changes in the brain chemistry after ECT, it is difficult to pinpoint the specific cause of relief.[23]

A full remission or marked improvement is reported in 90% of those treated. Another advantage of ECT is that improvement is rapid, whereas with medication there may be a four-to-twelve week period before the depression lifts completely. If a patient is suicidal, this period can be critical.[8, 9, 23]

Repetitive transcranial magnetic stimulation (TMS)

TMS uses a hand-held electrical coil that is placed on the scalp at the location of the left prefrontal cortex. An electrical current is passed through the coil, generating a magnetic pulse that passes through the skull and into the brain. It is believed that the electrical field this creates leads to a depolarization of neurons in the brain. Although the procedure is similar in some ways to ECT, no anesthesia is required. There is some concern that TMS might induce seizures, although so far none have been reported.[24]

Patients with treatment-resistant depression who were treated using TMS had a greater decrease in depressive symptoms than the control group, indicating that TMS has a role in medication-resistant depression. TMS is currently under FDA review.[24]

Vagus nerve stimulation (VNS)

The successful use of VNS as a treatment for epilepsy led to hope that it might also be an effective treatment for depression and bipolar disorder. The treatment costs $15,000 and up and requires surgery for the implantation of a battery-operated device in the upper left part of the chest. Tubes containing electrodes extend from the device and wrap around the vagus nerve at the point where it passes through the neck. The device delivers a mild electrical pulse every five minutes which lasts about 30 seconds. The battery needs to be replaced every five to ten years, which requires an additional surgery.

Patients who were not responsive to antidepressant medications were tested using VNS. After three months of treatment, 30% showed improvement; after a full year of treatment, 45% had improved, with 29% recovering completely. To date, no serious adverse effects from VNS have been observed. VNS is approved as a treatment for depression in the European Union, but not yet in the U.S.[25]

Direct Relevance to Psychotherapy

There are many different effective ways to intervene when a patient exhibits symptoms of depression. The efficacy of any specific intervention depends on many factors, both situational and personal. When the symptoms are severe, such as when a client is rapidly losing weight or is suicidal, quick relief is essential.

Most experts agree that depression has cognitive, affective, and vegetative components; intervention at any of these levels will affect the depression, and each type of intervention may have different results. Cognitive therapy, behavior modification, and psychoactive medications are all appropriate treatments for depression. Any or all of these may be necessary for optimal patient care. It is important that the therapist and the client collaborate to determine which treatment, or combination of treatments, is most appropriate, and whether a referral to a psychiatrist for medication is necessary.

Sometimes psychotherapists are reluctant to recommend that clients see a psychiatrist for a medication evaluation. Some therapists believe that medication should not be necessary in order to gain relief of symptoms. More often, it is the client who is averse to the idea of taking medication, and may have chosen treatment by a psychotherapist rather than by a psychiatrist specifically for this reason. It is not unusual that the most difficult aspect for the psychotherapist is the patient's resistance to taking medication. It is essential that these issues be explored as part of the psychotherapy.

In addition to their personal biases, both the therapist and the client may be concerned about the costs of a medication evaluation, the necessary lab tests, and the ongoing cost of the drug itself. Also entering into the calculus are the adverse effects and whether the potential good of taking a medication outweighs the possible harm.

While all of these reasons have some validity, there can be no doubt that the psychotherapist's primary consideration must be to objectively evaluate the facts so as to be able to support the optimal treatment for each client. The symptoms of depression can be severe, and the disease can be life-threatening, so it is essential that the psychotherapist has both an open mind and objective standards to help decide when a medication evaluation is necessary.

The assessment of the client's symptoms is readily available as a measure. Referral to a psychiatrist for medication is appropriate if symptoms are severe and have not lessened considerably after three weeks of psychotherapy. Severe symptoms include the presence of suicidal ideation, rapid loss of weight (more than 15 pounds), and an inability to perform normal activities at work, school, or in social settings.

A therapist may believe that taking medication interferes with the therapeutic process and prevents "working through" the underlying cause or causes of the depression. It is true that sometimes a depressed patient who is not on medication is unable to function in the world, yet when on medication cannot go very deeply into the therapy process. In this situation, the psychotherapist may conclude that the underlying dynamics will not be worked through. On rare occasions this does occur, but most often clients who are on medication are both more functional and more capable of doing their psychotherapeutic work. In some instances, a client's therapy deepens while on medication due to a decrease in apathy or anxiety, either of which may have been impeding motivation or access to information. A successful course of medication will allow the person to resume a more normal life; this raises the client's level of self-esteem, which in itself is therapeutic.

When a client is on medication, it is important for a good working relationship to exist between the psychotherapist and the psychiatrist. Since the therapist usually sees the client much more frequently than the psychiatrist does, the therapist will often be the first to notice changes and/or adverse effects. It is also important for psychotherapists to encourage clients to contact their psychiatrists if symptoms worsen or if no improvement is seen.

All antidepressant medications and ECT have significant adverse effects and should only be used when the depression is seriously debilitating. Both the immediate and long-term consequences must be considered. The determination as to whether any specific medication is appropriate requires the combined efforts of the psychiatrist—with expertise in medical assessment and experience with prescribing different drugs—in collaboration with the patient and the psychotherapist.

Often patients who are on antidepressants do not inform their psychiatrists that they are discontinuing their medication. The psychotherapist should frequently check with patients as to how they are feeling about their medication, whether they think it is helping, and whether they are still taking it. It is the responsibility of the psychotherapist to inform any client who is considering decreasing or stopping antidepressant medication that this must be done under the supervision of the psychiatrist in order to decrease the likelihood of a recurrence of depressive symptoms and other adverse effects.

Usually, after a patient with a first episode of depression has been asymptomatic for nine months to a year, the psychiatrist, psychotherapist, and patient will consult to determine if it is the right time to try eliminating the medication. If deemed appropriate, the psychiatrist will work with the patient to develop a schedule for slowly decreasing the dosage. If withdrawn too rapidly, a recurrence of depression is likely to occur, along with other symptoms such as nausea, vomiting, dizziness, chills, sweating, abdominal cramping, diarrhea, insomnia, irritability, and anxiety.

The risk of suicide in depressed patients is greatest four to five months after the symptoms have abated. This is because while in the depths of depression people do not usually have enough energy to commit suicide. If after feeling better for a while a patient's depression returns, he or she may lose all hope of ever being free of the disease. For this reason, it is advisable to continue medication for at least five months after the depression lifts. After that, the risk of suicide is greatly diminished.

The psychotherapist must always weigh the risks and the benefits of any type of treatment. Some clients are not able to do psychotherapy without medication, and some cannot do psychotherapy with it. You, as the psychotherapist, along with the client and the psychiatrist, will help to determine the most appropriate treatment. It is through collaboration and open communication that we can best serve our patients.

References for Chapter 4

1. Sheline, Y. I., Wang, P. W., Gado, M. H., Csernansky, J. G. & Vannier, M. W. (1996). Hippocampal atrophy in recurrent major depression. *Proc. Natl. Acad. Sci.*, USA 93, 3908–3913.
2. Keller, M. B., Lavori, P. W. & Mueller, T. I. (1992). Time to recovery, chronicity, and levels of psychopathology in major depression. *Arch. Gen. Psychiatry*, 49, 809–816.
3. American Psychiatric Association. (1994). *Diagnostic and statistical manual of mental disorders* (4th ed.). Wash., DC: American Psychiatric Association.
4. Kendler, K. S. & Prescott, C. A. (1999). A population-based twin study of lifetime major depression in men and women. *Arch. Gen. Psychiatry*, 56(1), 39–44.
5. National Institute of Mental Health (NIMH). Retrieved Sept. 1, 2003 from http://www.surgeongeneral.gov/library/mentalhealth/chapter4/sec3_1.html.
6. Oquendo, M. A., Malone, K. M. & Ellis, S. P. (1999). Inadequacy of antidepressant treatment for patients with major depression who are at risk for suicidal behavior. *Am. J. Psychiatry*, 156, 190–194.
7. Greden, J. F. (2001). Clinical prevention of recurrent depression, In: Greden, J. F., (Ed.) *Treatment of Recurrent Depression. Review of Psychiatry*, 20(5), 143–170. Washington, DC: American Psychiatric Publishing.
8. Fink, M. (2001). ECT has much to offer our patients: It should not be ignored. *World J. Biol. Psychiatry*, 2, 1–8.
9. Avery, D. & Lubrano, A. (1979). Depression treated with imipramine and ECT: The DeCarolis study reconsidered. *Am. J. Psychiatry*, 136, 559–562.
10. Fox-Aarons, S., Frances, A. J. & Mann, J. (1985). Atypical depression: A review of diagnosis and treatment. *Hospital and Community Psychiatry*, 36, 275–282.
11. Lane, R., Baldwin, D., & Preskorn, S. (1995). The SSRIs: Advantages, disadvantages and differences. *J Psychopharmacol.* 9(suppl), 163–178.
12. Clayton, A. H., Pradko, J. F. & Kroft, H. A. (2002). Prevalence of sexual dysfunction among newer antidepressants. *J. Clin. Psychiatry*, 63, 357–366.
13. Nurnberg, H. G., Laurello, J. & Hensley, P. L. (1999). Sildenafil for sexual dysfunction in women taking antidepressants. *Am. J. Psychiatry*, 156, 1664.
14. Diler, R. S., Yolga, A. & Avci, A. (2002). Fluoxetine-induced extrapyramidal

symptoms in an adolescent: A case report. *Swiss Med. Wkly.*, 132, 125–126.

15. Lane, R. & Baldwin, D. (1997). Selective serotonin reuptake inhibitor-induced serotonin syndrome. Review. *J. Clinical Psychopharm.*, 17(3), 208–221.

16. Manfredonia, Maria Grazia. (1997). *Psicofarmaci.* {Psychopharmacology} Milan, Italy: il Saggiatore/Flammarion.

17. Guelfi, J. D., Ansseau, M., Timmerman, L. & Korsgaard, S. (2001). Mirtazapine versus venlafaxine in hospitalized severely depressed patients with melancholic features. *J. Clin. Psychopharm.*, 20, 531–537.

18. Roose, S. P., Glassman, A. H., Giardina, E. G. V., Walsh, B. T., Woodring, S. & Bigger, J. T. (1987). Tricyclic antidepressants in depressed patients with cardiac conduction disease. *Arch. Gen. Psychiatry*, 44, 273–275.

19. Bodkin, J. A. & Amsterdam, J. D. (2002). Transdermal selegiline in major depression: A double-blind, placebo controlled, parallel-group study in outpatients. *Am. J. Psychiatry*, 159, 1869–1875.

20. Clayton, A. H., Warnock, J. K., Kornstein, S. G. (2004). A placebo-controlled trial of bupropion SR as an antidote for selective serotonin reuptake inhibitor-induced sexual dysfunction. *J. Clin. Psychiatry*, 65(1), 62–67.

21. Parker, G. (2002). Olanzapine augmentation in the treatment of melancholia: The trajectory of improvement in rapid responders. *Int. Clin. Psychopharm.*, 17, 87–89.

22. Mantyh, P. W. (2002). Neurobiology of substance P and the NK1 receptor. *J. Clinical Psychiatry*, 63(suppl. 11), 6–10.

23. Abrams, Richard, MD. (2002). *Electroconvulsive therapy.* NY: Oxford Univ. Press.

24. Kozel, F. A. & George, M. S. (2002). Meta-analysis of left frontal repetitive transcranial magnetic stimulation (rTMS) to treat depression. *J. Psychiatric Practice*, 8, 270–275.

25. Schachter S. C. (2002). Vagus nerve stimulation: Where are we? *Current Opinion in Neurology*, 15(2), 201–206.

Chapter 5
Treatment of Bipolar Disorder

The suicide rate for people with untreated bipolar disorder is about 30 times greater than for the general population.[1] Studies show that people with bipolar disorder see an average of three to four doctors and spend more than eight years seeking treatment before getting a correct diagnosis. There are strong indications of a genetic component; children of a person with bipolar disorder have one chance in seven of also developing it.[2] Diagnosing children 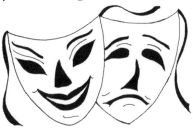 with bipolar disorder is very difficult because the symptoms they present are not the same as those seen in adults.

Between two and ten million Americans suffer from bipolar disorder. In adults, it is typically distinguished by a characteristic fluctuation between manic and depressed moods, often with no apparent cause for the shift. Most patients find their depressed moods unpleasant and want them to stop, whereas because it is usually experienced as an invigorating "high," they often want the manic state to continue. In contrast, friends, relatives, and therapists usually support whatever measures are necessary to end a manic state. These "outsiders" have too often seen bipolar sufferers getting into severe work, financial, and relationship difficulties due to their behaviors when not on medication. The primary reason many bipolar patients repeatedly cycle in and out of mental hospitals is their unsupervised discontinuance of medication.

Examples of manic behavior
Some typical examples of manic behaviors are:

- restlessness
- argumentativeness
- sexual promiscuity
- no desire for sleep
- out of control gambling
- effusive/expansive mood
- excessive spending/talking[3]

It is known that life-stressors, such as substance abuse or lack of sleep, can trigger a manic episode. Mood swings become more frequent during periods without treatment. On average, there are four episodes of mania or depression in the first 10 years of illness. These episodes can last for days, months, or even years. Without treatment, the depression usually lasts about six months, while the manic episodes are generally shorter, usually a few months. Some people recover completely between episodes, while others have milder but continuing symptoms of mania or depression.

Cognitive deficits

Some patients with bipolar disorder exhibit cognitive deficits, particularly problems with memory. There is some evidence that taking the ACh inhibitors rivastigmine and galantamine may improve cognitive performance in these patients.[4]

Drugs Used to Treat Bipolar Disorder

LITHIUM

The active ingredient in the longest-used medication for the treatment of bipolar disorder is lithium (Li), the third element on the *Periodic Table of Elements*.[5] Lithium prevents manic episodes, and is somewhat useful in preventing relapses of depression. It works best for treating bipolar illness rather than for depressive disorders. It is not the first drug of choice for depression.

Sometimes patients treated with lithium alone have breakthrough episodes of depression (the depression "breaks through" the preventative treatment). If this occurs, most psychiatrists prescribe antidepressant medication in addition to the lithium, though usually on a short-term basis (on average for four to five months), and only when the depressive symptoms are present.[6,7] When the depression abates, most psychiatrists taper the patient off the antidepressant.

Effects of lithium

There is usually a lag period of four to ten days from the start of the medication for the antimanic effects to be seen. Behaviors exhibited during a manic episode can be dangerous, and for this reason while waiting for the antimanic effects of the lithium, a patient may be started on a sedating antipsychotic medication to quiet the agitation.[7] Antipsychotic medication is then slowly tapered off as lithium takes effect (generally one to two weeks). After that, antipsychotic medication is usually not necessary and is discontinued.[1]

Lithium has no observable effect on the mood of people who do not have bipolar disorder. It does not cause sedation or euphoria, so it is not likely to be abused. A person taking lithium who is dehydrated due to exercising vigorously or perspiring in hot weather is at a risk of overdose. Under these conditions, the concentration of lithium in the blood will increase; high levels can lead to a comatose state. Blood levels of patients on lithium must be carefully monitored, particularly if they are on low-salt diets, since this can lead to a loss of water in the body which will cause the blood levels of lithium to increase.[6]

Between 70% to 90% of bipolar disorder sufferers respond well to lithium, although it may take months to find the correct dose.[7] This lag in response time is one reason why the psychotherapist and the prescribing psychiatrist need to have a good collegial relationship. During this period, the therapist will need to provide the psychiatrist with feedback as to how the patient is responding to medication, since bipolar patients are often not the best judges of whether their level of medication is appropriate.

Adverse effects of lithium

Taking lithium can cause many adverse effects, including:

Kidney damage: When taken over long periods of time, lithium may cause serious kidney damage. For this reason, it is important for these patients to be carefully monitored by a medical doctor/psychiatrist. If kidney damage does occur, the patient must be taken off lithium and switched to another drug to control the manic behavior.[6, 8, 9]

Thyroid functioning: Lithium inhibits thyroid functioning. If hypothyroidism develops in response to lithium, it is usually remedied by prescribing thyroid hormone. If lithium is taken long-term, hypothyroidism will occur in approximately 15% of patients.[6] Irregularities in thyroid functioning may lead to either hyperactive or depressive symptoms. This effect can be clinically confusing since symptoms of hypothyroidism are similar to those of depression (lab tests may be required to differentiate between these two conditions). To rule out thyroid problems as an underlying cause of these symptoms, many psychiatrists require a thyroid panel. Thyroid functioning returns to normal when lithium is discontinued.[6]

Altered glucose metabolism: Lithium alters glucose tolerance, the complex process of glucose metabolism that regulates the absorption of glucose into blood and tissues via the insulin mechanism. Even patients who are not diabetic can develop a condition of mild diabetes while taking lithium. A person known to be diabetic before starting lithium requires careful monitoring to determine whether an adjustment in the usual dose of insulin is needed. The prescribing psychiatrist must carefully monitor medical conditions, and make adjustments as required, in the levels of lithium and/or hormones.[6]

ANTICONVULSANT MEDICATIONS FOR BIPOLAR DISORDER

Anticonvulsant medications are often used for the treatment of bipolar disorder for patients who do not respond to lithium, or for patients who are allergic to lithium or cannot tolerate its adverse effects. About 30% of people with bipolar disorder fall into one of these categories.[8]

Even though most are not FDA-approved as a maintenance treatment for bipolar disorder, many anticonvulsant drugs are used to control manic symptoms. Anticonvulsant drugs, in combination with lithium, are also used for patients whose manic symptoms do not abate with lithium alone. These drugs (particularly carbamazepine/Tegretol, valproate/Depakote, and gabapentin/Neurontin) are useful in treatment of acute manic states because they take effect more quickly than lithium.[9] Valproate has FDA-approval for its primary use as an antiseizure medication and also for the treatment of acute manic episodes.[8] These medications are less effective than lithium in preventing depressive episodes.[7]

Adverse effects of anticonvulsant drugs

The main danger in the use of anticonvulsants is that they can have the paradoxical effect of inducing a seizure if the dose is raised too quickly. Taking anticonvulsant drugs may also worsen any cardiac conduction disease already present (although these drugs are less cardiotoxic than TCAs and HCAs).[9]

Most of the anticonvulsant drugs are not useful for the treatment of the depressive aspect of bipolar disorder.

Teratogenic effects (birth defects)

There is some evidence that if taken during pregnancy valproate or carbamazepine may cause fetal malformations. Women taking antiseizure medications need to be informed about possible teratogenic effects. A recent study done in Finland found major malformations (neural tube defects, oral clefts, cardiovascular and visceral malformations) at a rate 14 times greater than in the rest of the Finnish population. Drugs taken by the women included valproate, carbamazepine, and oxcarbazepine. Women with epilepsy who were not taking antiseizure medication had a rate of fetal malformations similar to the rates seen in other women.[10]

Anticonvulsant Medications

- carbamazepine/Carbatrol, Tegretol
- gabapentin/Neurontin
- lamotrigine/Lamictal
- topiramate/Topamax
- valproate/Depakene, Depakote

Table 5.1

Effects on male reproductive function

Carbamazepine, oxcarbazepine and valproate have been found to be associated with sperm abnormalities. Valproate-treated men had both abnormal sperm and reduced testicular volume.[11]

Carbamazepine, adverse effects

Carbamazepine/Tegretol can cause serious hematological disturbances such as *aplastic anemia* (a decrease in all types of blood cells) and *agranulocytosis* (a decrease in the type of white blood cells called granulocytes). These blood disorders are seen in about one in every 20,000 patients treated. Aplastic anemia and agranulocytosis occur with about equal frequency.[12] Both conditions can be fatal. During the first few weeks of use, carbamazepine sometimes causes *hepatitis* (inflammation of the liver). This condition can be fatal if the hepatitis is not detected early and if the drug is continued. Carbamazepine can cause:

- nausea
- gastric distress
- vomiting
- anorexia
- diarrhea
- constipation[12]

Gabapentin, adverse effects

Since gabapentin/Neurontin is sedating, it is often chosen for patients who are more agitated or have ongoing sleep difficulties. Taking gabapentin can cause:

- sleepiness
- dizziness
- fatigue
- nausea
- vomiting
- unsteadiness

Valproate (divalproax sodium, valproic acid), adverse effects

The side effects of valproate/Depakene/Depakote are similar to other anticonvulsants. Tolerance to these effects usually develops after a few weeks. Blood disorders that result in prolongation of bleeding time also have been observed. There are other serious, adverse effects involving the pancreas and liver. Rare but serious cases of pancreatitis (inflammation of the pancreas) occasionally resulting in death have been reported.[8] Taking valproate can also cause:

- vomiting
- weight gain
- nausea
- hair loss
- sedation
- tremor[8]

A recent study compared the medical records of 20,638 patients with bipolar disorder who were taking either lithium or valproate. The researchers found that the patients taking valproate were 2.7 times more likely to kill themselves than those taking lithium. This study indicates that lithium should be considered the first drug of choice for the treatment of bipolar disorder.[13]

NEWER ANTICONVULSANT DRUGS

Lamotrigine

Lamotrigine/Lamictal, an antiseizure drug, is being recommended for bipolar maintenance and for the prevention of the recurrent depressive episodes that occur with this disorder. The main adverse effect of this drug is that it can cause a serious allergic reaction known as Stevens-Johnson Syndrome (SJS), a toxic epidermal necrosis. SJS occurs most frequently when the dose is increased rapidly. It occurs in one in 1,000 adults and in as many as 1% to 2% of children.[12] This effect can usually be alleviated by decreasing the dose. Generally, the dosage can be increased later without the symptoms returning.

Topiramate

Yet another antiseizure drug, topiramate/Topamax, is now being used as a mood stabilizer to treat bipolar disorder (although not FDA-approved for this use). Like most other antiseizure drugs, it is useful in controlling manic episodes and has the advantage of taking effect more quickly than lithium.[9] Weight loss has occurred in up to 90% of patients. This effect may be dose-related. As much as 7% of body weight has been lost in higher dose ranges (600 to 1000mg/day). Depending on the individual, the weight-loss may be regarded as positive or negative. There is evidence that topiramate is also effective in treating and preventing cluster headaches.[14]

The most common adverse effects of topiramate are:

- speech or language problems
- dizziness or balance problems
- feeling sluggish, sedated, confused
- feelings of being unusually tired or weak
- irregular eye movements and double-vision
- oligohidrosis (excessive sweating and hyperthermia), especially in pediatric patients[9]
- memory difficulties • nervousness • tremor

ANTIPSYCHOTIC MEDICATIONS FOR MANIA

The FDA has approved the antipsychotic drug olanzapine/Zyprexa for acute mania and bipolar maintenance.[15] Prior to this, various antipsychotic medications, since they are sedating, have been used without FDA approval to treat mania. These drugs have the advantage of controlling manic symptoms more rapidly than lithium. Sedation is usually immediate, and general improvement can be seen one week after the start of medication. These drugs may also be useful for people who cannot tolerate either lithium or anticonvulsants.

Risperidone and quetiapine have also been approved for the treatment of acute mania.[16, 17] Applications have also been filed with the FDA for the use of aripiprazole and ziprasidone for the treatment of acute mania.

Olanzapine and fluoxetine have been combined in a new compound called Symbyax which has been approved for the treatment of bipolar depression.

Direct Relevance to Psychotherapy

Most therapists agree that it is not possible to do psychotherapy with a client who is in a manic state. People in a manic state usually do not perceive problems with their behavior or feelings; therefore they do not see any need for medication or treatment. Paranoid delusions are often present, making it difficult to create and maintain a therapeutic alliance. Before effective psychotherapy can take place, the manic episode must be terminated.

There is evidence the use of cognitive therapy (CT), when used as an adjunct to medication, significantly reduces the rate of relapse for bipolar I patients. In one study, therapists taught their clients how to monitor for prodromal symptoms of relapse, to maintain regular schedules, and to moderate their attempts to compensate for the time they lost from work when feeling ill. Compared to control subjects, patients receiving CT had better medication compliance, better social functioning, fewer manic swings, and fewer hospitalizations.[18]

All antimanic drugs have adverse effects that can be serious and sometimes fatal.[12] It is very likely that psychotherapists, because they usually have more frequent contact with clients than psychiatrists, will be the first to recognize a serious adverse effect due to medication. For this reason, a collaborative relationship between the therapist and the prescribing psychiatrist is crucial when treating patients with bipolar disorder.

References for Chapter 5

1. Kahn, D. A., Ross, R., Rush, A. J. & Panico, S. (1996). Expert consensus guidelines for bipolar disorder: A guide for patients and families. *J. Clin. Psychiatry*, 57(suppl. 12A), 81–88.
2. Kendler, K. S. & Prescott, C. A. (1999). A population-based twin study of lifetime major depression in men and women. *Arch. Gen. Psychiatry*, Jan., 56(1), 39–44.
3. American Psychiatric Association. (1994). *Diagnostic and statistical manual of mental disorders* (4th ed). Wash., DC: American Psychiatric Association.
4. Hussain, M. Z., Chaudry, Z. A. & Hussain, S. (2003). Rivastigmine tartrate and galant-

amine in neurocognitive deficits in bipolar mood disorder. *156th Annual meeting of the American Psychiatric Association*, May, 2003, San Francisco.

5. Periodic Table of the elements, retrieved Oct. 12, 2003, from http://www.webelements.com/

6. Bowden, C. L. (1998). Key treatment studies of lithium in manic-depressive illness: Efficacy and side effects. *J. Clin. Psychiatry*, 59(suppl. 6), 13–20.

7. Baldessarini, R. J., Tondo, L., Hennen, J. & Viguera, A. C. (2002). Is lithium still worth using? An update of selected recent research. *Harvard Rev. Psychiatry*, 10, 59–75.

8. Pope, H. G. Jr., Mc Elroy, S. L., Keck, P. E. Jr. & Hudson, J. I. (1991). Valproate in the treatment of acute mania: A placebo controlled study. *Arch. Gen. Psychiatry*, 48, 62–68.

9. Dunn, R. T., Frye, M. S., Kimbrell, T. A., Denicoff, K. D., Leverich, G. S. & Post, R. M. (1998). The efficacy and use of anticonvulsants in mood disorders. *Clinical Neuropharm.*, 21, 215–235.

10. Kaaja, E (2003). Fetal malformations. *Neurology*, 60, 575–579.

11. Isojarvi, J. I., Lofgren, E., Juntunen, K. S., Pakarinen, A. J., Paivansalo, M., Rautakorpi, I. & Tuomivaara, L. (2004). Effect of epilepsy and antiepileptic drugs on male reproductive health. *Neurology*, 62, 247–253.

12. *The Merck manual of diagnosis and therapy*. (2001) (17th ed.). Rahway, NJ: Merck Sharp & Dohme Research Laboratories.

13. Goodwin, F. K., Fireman, B., Simon, G. E., Hunkeler, E. M., Lee, J. & Revicki, D. (2003). Suicide risk in bipolar disorder during treatment with lithium and divalproex. *JAMA*, 290(11), 1467–1473.

14. Lainez, M. J., Pascual, J., Pascual, A. M., Santonja, J. M., Ponz, A. & Salvador, A. (2003). Topiramate in the prophylactic treatment of cluster headache. *Headache*, 43, 784–789.

15. Tohen, M., Sanger, T. M., McElroy, S. L., Tollefson, G. D., Royu-Chenappa, K. N., Daniel, D. G., Petty, F., Centorrino, F., Wang, R., Grundy, S. L., Greaney, M. G., Jacobs, T. G., David, S. R. & Toma, V., (1999). Olanzapine versus placebo in the treatment of acute mania. *Am. J. Psychiatry*, 156, 702–709.

16. Guille, C., Sachs, G. S. & Ghaemi, S. N. (2000). A naturalistic comparison of clozapine, risperidone, and olanzapine in the treatment of bipolar disorder. *J. Clin. Psychiatry*, 61, 638–642.

17. Ghaemi, S. N. & Sachs, G. S. (1997). Long term risperidone treatment in bipolar disorder: 6-month follow up. *Int. Clin. Psychopharmacol.*, 12, 333–338.

18. Lam, D. H. (2003). Cognitive therapy for relapse prevention for bipolar disorder. *Arch. Gen. Psych.*, 60, 145–152.

Chapter 6

CNS Stimulants: Use & Abuse

I love coffee, I love tea
I love the java jive and it loves me
Coffee and tea and the jivin' and me
A cup, a cup, a cup, a cup, a cup!
"Java Jive," 1940

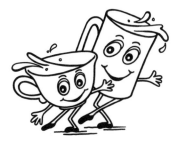

The class of drugs designated as central nervous system (CNS) stimulants includes the two most frequently-used drugs on the planet, caffeine and nicotine. This class also includes the amphetamines, cocaine, and methylphenidate/Ritalin.

General Effects of Stimulants

All stimulant drugs cause an increase in general behavioral activity. When taken short-term (one or two weeks), stimulant drugs cause states of euphoria, optimism, and general feelings of well-being. Initial feelings of anorexia are frequent with stimulants, a quality that leads to their use/abuse in diet formulations. Insomnia is another common effect. These responses indicate that the part of the brain which controls these functions, the hypothalamus, is strongly affected. Other effects are:

- anxiety
- irritability
- decreased fatigue
- increased talkativeness
- increased blood pressure
- decreased feelings of depression
- increased thoughts and associations

Tolerance to stimulants

Tolerance to the mood-elevating and appetite-suppressing effects develops after about two weeks of daily use. Little tolerance develops to the behavioral-arousal effect, which is what makes these drugs useful in the long-term treatment of narcolepsy.[1]

Abuse of Stimulants & Treatments for Withdrawal

A person who is addicted to stimulants, or who has had a long period of continuous use, will experience withdrawal symptoms if the drug is stopped abruptly. Symptoms of withdrawal from amphetamines and cocaine are very similar, mainly feelings of depression, fatigue, apathy, and general sluggishness—the opposite of effects seen under the influence of these drugs. These symptoms, though not physically dangerous, can be extremely uncomfortable.[2]

If a depressed person has been using stimulants on a long-term basis, has become dependent, or is abusing these drugs and increasing the dosage, then a severe depression may occur when the drug is withdrawn.[2] If the depression caused by withdrawal does not abate after a week or two, evaluation by a psychiatrist for antidepressant medication is appropriate.

AMPHETAMINES

Amphetamine, dextroamphetamine, and methamphetamine (collectively referred to as "amphetamines") all have very similar properties. The first amphetamine was synthesized in 1887, but it was not until the 1920's that it was investigated as a treatment for a variety of ills such as depression and decongestion. In the 1930's, an inhaler under the name Benzedrine was sold over-the-counter and marketed for the treatment of asthma, hay fever, and the common cold. Methamphetamine, discovered in 1919, is a crystalline powder that is easy to make (this is the "speed," "crank," or "meth" often made in illegal drug labs) and can be injected when dissolved in water. During World War II, amphetamines were sometimes used to push soldiers to their limits, and even today "go pills" are used by U.S. military pilots. Dextroamphetamine/Dexedrine and methamphetamine/Methedrine were widely available in the 1950's and used by truck drivers and college students to stay awake, by athletes to enhance performance,[3] and by millions as an appetite suppressant.

Ondansetron for amphetamine withdrawal

The antinausea drug ondansetron/Zofran has been found to stop cravings in early-onset alcoholics, and is now being tested as an aid for abstinence for those addicted to methamphetamine. Habitual users are unable to get high while taking it. It appears to work by enhancing 5-HT transmission.[4]

COCAINE

Evidence suggests that the coca plant, *Erythroxylum coca,* was domesticated in South America around 1500 BCE. To this day, coca is an important part of many cultures in the Andes, where it is used in social rituals and its leaves are chewed to provide stimulation and relief from hunger. The plant's active ingredient, cocaine, was isolated by chemists in 1860. In the latter half of the 19th century, cocaine was considered to be an elixir, and was included in many patent medicines. Coca-Cola®, which takes its name from the coca plant, included cocaine as an ingredient when it was introduced in 1885, which helped to make Coke® the world's most popular soft drink. The cocaine was removed in 1903 as its dangers began to be recognized.[5]

Cocaine ("coke," "crack") is a potent CNS stimulant which is bio-chemically similar to the amphetamines and produces similar (although shorter-lasting) mood-elevating effects. The behavioral effects of cocaine are also similar to those of the amphetamines. Cocaine in various forms (Novocaine, Lidocaine, Carbocaine) has been used as a local anesthetic for many years.

A medicinal concoction of cocaine, methadone, and alcohol, called "Brompton's cocktail," is sometimes given to terminally-ill patients in extreme pain. Brompton's cocktail is not used more generally because it has the potential to be highly addictive due to the rapid onset of both stimulant and euphoric effects.

Treatment for cocaine withdrawal

Recreational use of cocaine can be lethal, particularly if taken by injection. Fatality can result from heart failure, respiratory depression, stroke, or seizures.[2] In terms of psychological effects, cocaine use can produce a psychosis that is indistinguishable from one seen with paranoid schizophrenia. Physical dependence has not been demonstrated, although there is evidence that a very strong psychological dependence can develop.[2]

Some treatments for cocaine withdrawal are based on the belief that many people use stimulant drugs to self-medicate a depressive disorder. It is thought that people suffering from depressive disorders may not have enough endogenous NE and 5-HT, and they use stimulants to increase the amounts of neuromodulator available. In support of this theory are the positive results seen when the antidepressant desipramine/Norpramin (a TCA) is taken at the time of stimulant withdrawal. Desipramine works by inhibiting reuptake of NE, which results in an increase in NE at the synapse. This leads to an increase in neuronal stimulation and increased feelings of energy. Patients taking an antidepressant medication may be less likely to use cocaine to ward off depression.

Psychotic symptoms in cocaine withdrawal

A treatment dilemma may occur if the cocaine user is also having psychotic symptoms and needs to be treated with an antipsychotic drug. Administration of antipsychotic drugs leads to an increased craving for cocaine, which may in turn lead to an increase in drug use, which then may lead to a worsening of psychotic symptoms.[2]

Gamma-vinyl-GABA (GVG) for cocaine withdrawal

GVG is an antiepileptic drug which has been shown to reduce cocaine cravings. It is believed to work by increasing the amount of GABA in the CNS. The usual side effects are sleepiness and fatigue. It is not approved for use in the U.S. but is available in Canada and other countries.[6]

Disulfiram treatment for cocaine dependence

Disulfiram has been evaluated as a treatment for individuals with comorbid alcohol and cocaine abuse. Disulfiram-treated subjects decreased the quantity and frequency of their cocaine use significantly more than those treated with placebo.[7]

Gabapentin for cocaine dependence

Gabapentin/Neurontin is an antiepileptic drug which appears to be safe and effective in reducing cocaine usage.[8]

Modafinil for cocaine dependence

One study compared the use of cognitive behavioral therapy to a combination of cognitive behavioral therapy and modafinil with subjects in recovery for cocaine use. Those subjects receiving both modafinil and CBT were more likely to remain cocaine-free than those receiving CBT alone.[9]

Cocaine vaccine

A vaccine is being tested that induces the formation of anticocaine antibodies. The antibodies combine with cocaine to form a large molecular complex that has difficulty crossing the blood-brain barrier, which decreases the amount of cocaine that can get into the brain. If only a small amount of cocaine gets into the brain, the impact on the pleasure centers is greatly diminished. In animal models, addiction was extinguished using these methods. The antibodies remain in the blood and are effective for six months to one year, after which booster shots might be required. One danger with this treatment is that very large doses of cocaine might be able to overcome the antibodies; this could lead to a lethal overdose. It is expected that the vaccine will be a valuable adjunct to psychotherapy for cocaine users who want to overcome their addiction.[10]

Relapse Prevention therapy/Harm-Reduction model

Relapse Prevention therapy (RP) (also known as the Harm-Reduction model) is one of the few scientifically validated psychosocial treatments for substance abuse and has been proven useful for treatment of cocaine abuse. No other type of treatment is without major difficulties or side effects. RP techniques help people recognize high-risk situations, rehearse ways to deal with them, self-monitor substance use, and learn to deal with cravings by understanding and discussing them. With this type of therapy, lapses in behavior are regarded as learning tools (i.e., ways to understand what happened) as well as opportunities to renew the commitment to sobriety. RP does not result in greater abstinence rates than other treatments, but relapses are shorter and less frequent. RP may be better in the long term for maintaining a lower relapse rate because over time people continue to improve as they practice avoiding relapse.[11, 12]

CAFFEINE

Coffee and tea are the most common sources of caffeine. Tea is made from the leaves of the *Camellia sinensis* plant, and is believed to have been in use in China since about 2700 BCE. The legend is that a servant of the emperor was boiling water when the leaf of an overhead tree dropped into the water, and the emperor decided to taste it.[13]

Coffee is made from the berries of a species of the genus *Coffea*, in particular *Coffea arabica* and *Coffea canephora*. One legend says that its stimulant property was discovered by a shepherd who observed his flock becoming hyperactive after eating the bright red berries. Coffee has been consumed as a beverage in Middle Eastern cultures

since about 1100 CE. When it was introduced to
Europe in about 1600, many considered it the
"devil's drink" because it was popular in non-
Christian societies. Then the pope tried it, and he
liked it so much he "baptized" it, removing its alien
stigma.[14]

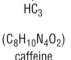

$(C_8H_{10}N_4O_2)$
caffeine

Fig. 6.1

Caffeine is the most widely-used psychoactive
substance. Eighty-nine percent of adults in North
America use either coffee or caffeinated tea daily. The average coffee
drinker consumes approximately 1,000 cups per year, or about three
cups per day. Most people do not think of it as a drug, but caffeine
is a powerful stimulant, and although its use is legal, overdosing on
caffeine (more than 5 to 10 grams at one time) can be fatal. Caffeine
is quite addicting; a tolerance and tendency to increase intake are
common, and withdrawal symptoms will occur if consumption is
stopped.[15]

Because caffeine makes people feel better in general, it is often
included as an ingredient in analgesics (e.g. Anacin, Excedrin) as well
as in many cold preparations. Caffeine intake can be estimated using
Table 6.1 (p. 85). Keep in mind that caffeine content varies depending on the product used and the method of preparation.

Effects of caffeine

Caffeine causes an increase in cellular activity in the CNS and
behavioral and emotional responses that are similar to, but milder than,
the amphetamines and cocaine. After consuming caffeine, people
report thinking more clearly, having more energy, and having faster
reaction times.[15] Increases are seen in respiratory rate, amplitude of
reflexes, and the rate and force of the heart's contractions (systolic
pressure).

Caffeine causes a general *vasodilatation* (opening) of the systemic
blood vessels, including the coronary arteries, resulting in an increase
in blood-flow to the heart. Duration of systemic vasodilatation is brief

and is accompanied by *vasoconstriction* (tightening) of the vessels in the brain.[15] Central vasoconstriction is the mechanism by which caffeine provides relief from both hypertensive and migraine headaches (another reason why caffeine is often found in headache remedies).

Caffeine dependence

People who are caffeine-dependent have a strong association between caffeine consumption and feelings of well-being. Many people enjoy the increased speed of performance and feelings of efficiency caused by caffeine. Regular caffeine consumption causes both psychological dependence and physiological tolerance.[15]

Caffeinism

This disorder is a chronic toxicity caused by high levels of caffeine consumption. It is characterized by:

- disruption of sleep patterns
- nausea
- diarrhea
- headache
- trembling
- dry mouth
- palpitations
- depression
- stomach pain
- feelings of anxiety
- ringing in the ears
- irregular heartbeat
- rapid changes in mood

Caffeine withdrawal

The main symptom is headaches; these may continue for up to five days if no caffeine is consumed. The headaches often lead the sufferer to use analgesic preparations which may contain caffeine. This will cure the headache, but will lead to a continuance of caffeine dependence. Other symptoms of caffeine withdrawal are:

- apathy
- irritability
- restlessness
- decreased efficiency
- lethargy
- mild nausea
- nervousness
- difficulty concentrating

It is possible to reduce withdrawal symptoms by gradually decreasing the daily intake of caffeine by substituting decaffeinated coffee for regular and increasing the percentage of decaf each day.

Other effects of caffeine

Even though no significant correlation between birth defects and caffeine consumption has yet been demonstrated, it is important for women to know that caffeine crosses the placenta and gets into the bloodstream of a developing fetus. It also gets into the breast milk of nursing mothers. In both cases, the fetus or infant is ingesting a portion of the caffeine consumed by its mother.

Caffeine Content		
SOURCE	SERVING	CAFFEINE* (mg)
coffee (drip)	8 oz.	175–240
coffee (perked)	8 oz.	100–200
coffee (instant)	8 oz.	65–170
coffee (decaffeinated)	8 oz.	3–8
black tea (steeped 5 min.)	8 oz.	65–160
green tea (steeped 5 min.)	8 oz.	80
hot cocoa	8 oz.	3–16
cola beverages	12 oz.	45
"energy" beverages	8 oz.	80
milk chocolate	1 oz.	1–15
bittersweet chocolate	1 oz.	3–35
chocolate cake	1 slice	20–30
Anacin, Midol	2 tablets	64
Excedrin	2 tablets	130
NoDoz	2 tablets	200
Dexatrim	2 tablets	200
* Food & beverage contents approximate.		Table 6.1

There seems to be some relationship between caffeine and *fibrocystic breast disease*, although the specifics are not yet clearly understood.[15] Decreasing caffeine consumption leads to a decrease in discomfort experienced by women this disease. Many studies have been done with large numbers of adults, and no correlation between caffeine consumption and cancer has been substantiated.

One factor that reflects a physiological change to caffeine is age. People become more sensitive to caffeine's effects as they get older. It has also been observed that the amount of caffeine in the bloodstream increases when tobacco smoking is stopped. This increase in the blood level of caffeine will amplify the usual effects of nicotine withdrawal, such as irritability, nervousness, an inability to concentrate, and sleeplessness.

Studies show a positive correlation between caffeine use and anxiety disorders. People with anxiety disorders have an increased sensitivity to caffeine.[16] Symptoms of anxiety decrease with caffeine abstention, and for some people antianxiety medication is not necessary if caffeine use is discontinued.[17] The psychotherapist needs to assess caffeine intake in any patient who presents with symptoms of anxiety.

NICOTINE

The source of nicotine is the tobacco plant, *Nicotiana tabacum,* which is native to the western hemisphere. Tobacco was used by indigenous peoples throughout the Americas when the first explorers arrived from Europe, and its use quickly spread to the Old World.[18]

Today, nicotine is widely used in almost every country. Over 25% of American adults (about 50 million people) use tobacco products.[19] Although nicotine is extremely addictive, its purchase and use by anyone over the age of 18 is legal. If one considers how difficult it is to stop using it, nicotine is even more addictive than opioids. Using nicotine, particularly through smoking, is much more harmful than many other drugs in terms of number of illnesses it causes, the costs of treating those illnesses, and the high fatality rates among habitual users. While antismoking campaigns have lowered smoking rates in the U.S., the percentage of people worldwide who smoke is increasing. It is estimated there are more than 430,000 smoking-related deaths every year in the U.S. alone.[20]

Although nicotine is the ingredient in tobacco that causes physical dependency, it is the "tars" that contain the carcinogens. Nicotine consumption causes the release of NE, DA, and 5-HT in the CNS. This leads to feelings of both stimulation and calming. Research indicates that part of the calming effect experienced by smokers is due to the decrease in the unpleasant withdrawal symptoms a habitual user experiences as nicotine levels in the blood drop. When nonsmokers or former smokers are compared to current smokers, indications are that nicotine is not calming but actually increases stress.[21]

Effects of nicotine

The release of DA is probably what leads to the reinforcing experience of pleasure associated with tobacco (this is similar to other addictive drugs). Nicotine has a half-life of 30 minutes, which leads to an urge to consume more nicotine every half hour. Two cigarettes an hour (or consuming the equivalent form of other tobacco products) maintains a constant blood level of nicotine.

Tobacco leaf
Nicotiana tabacum

For reasons that are not yet clear, about 10% of people who smoke do not become addicted. They are able to keep consumption of cigarettes to approximately five per day, as opposed to the one or two packs a day consumed by the addict.[22] MRI and PET scans of drug abusers show that heightened craving is linked to increased activity in the frontal cortex. Research indicates that drug users who do not have decision-making impairment may have a lower risk for becoming addicted. This provides evidence that addiction may also be related to a disruption to motivational circuits in the CNS rather than only to pleasure-control centers.[4] These findings may help to explain why some drug users become addicted while others do not and may lead to better intervention strategies.

People who are addicted to nicotine have higher rates of major depression and anxiety disorders than people who smoke but do not become addicted.[23] One recent study found that 90% of people who attempt suicide are smokers.[24] More research is needed to determine the factors responsible for these differences.

It is estimated that about 70% of people with schizophrenia

smoke, a much higher percentage than in the general population. There is evidence that cigarette smoking ameliorates the unpleasant symptoms caused by schizophrenia and by antipsychotic medication. Atypical antipsychotic drugs (e.g. risperidone, olanzapine) have been shown to reduce cigarette smoking. The harm-reduction approach is the recommended method of treatment for decreasing the use of cigarettes in this population. The use of the nicotine patch or chewing gum, along with bupropion (see below), is recommended for maintenance treatment.[25]

Tars & other compounds found in tobacco products

Some known carcinogens found in tobacco tars include:

- benzopyrenes
- aromatic amines
- pyrenes
- chrysenes
- nitrosamines

There are many other substances known to be harmful to humans that are frequently present in tobacco products, including:

- cresols
- phenols
- metallic ions
- radioactive compounds
- carboxylic acids
- various additives and flavoring agents
- agricultural compounds (e.g., pesticides)

If manufacturers removed these toxic agents from their products the harmful effects of tobacco use would be greatly reduced.

Nicotine withdrawal

Physiological symptoms of withdrawal occur when someone who is addicted to nicotine stops consuming it. This withdrawal syndrome is commonly called a "nicotine fit." Some of the symptoms of nicotine withdrawal are:

- anxiety
- restlessness
- feelings of uneasiness
- headache
- nervousness
- digestive disturbances
- impairment of psychomotor performance
- impairment of concentration and judgement

When the body is under stress, nicotine is depleted faster than usual, causing the addict to increase consumption in order to maintain the usual blood-level of nicotine and to ward off symptoms of withdrawal.

Bupropion & naltrexone for nicotine withdrawal

The FDA's Drug Abuse Advisory Council found that the antidepressant bupropion/Wellbutrin/Zyban is safe and effective as an aid in smoking cessation.[26] The drug naltrexone/ReVia, developed for use during opioid withdrawal, has also been found to decrease the craving for nicotine. Both of these drugs are helpful as supportive measures in addition to psychotherapy, especially in the early stages of abstinence.

Clonidine for nicotine withdrawal

Another drug that helps with nicotine withdrawal is clonidine/Catapres. Clonidine is an antihypertensive drug that stimulates endorphin production; this leads to an increase in positive feelings. The craving for cigarettes is decreased if clonidine is taken during nicotine withdrawal.[27]

Gamma-vinyl-GABA for nicotine withdrawal

The antiepilepsy drug gamma vinyl-GABA/GVG is being tested to decrease nicotine-craving during withdrawal. GVG inhibits release of DA and increases production of GABA. The increased GABA would cause a calming effect.[28]

Patches, gums, lozenges & inhalers for tobacco withdrawal

The nicotine patch, nicotine gum, nicotine lozenges or a nicotine inhaler are all useful for helping people to decrease tobacco use and quit. Simply trying to "cut down" continues to expose the client to the health risks and reinforcing behaviors inherent in tobacco use. These products contain nicotine and are addictive.

Effect of caffeine during nicotine withdrawal

Caffeine is metabolized more quickly by smokers than by nonsmokers. If someone stops using nicotine, and the amount of caffeine consumed remains constant, the level of caffeine in the blood will double. This will cause an increase in nervousness that makes withdrawal from nicotine even more difficult. For this reason, it is recommended that caffeine consumption be decreased or eliminated during withdrawal from nicotine.[17]

Stimulants for Treatment of ADHD

Using the *DSM-IV* definition, the prevalence of *attention deficit hyperactivity disorder* (ADHD) in the U.S. is between 8% and 16%. Boys are four times more likely to be given this diagnosis than are girls.[29]

Amphetamines & methylphenidate/Ritalin

Methylphenidate was synthesized in the 1940's and marketed under the brand name Ritalin in the 1960's.[30] About 11 million prescriptions are written every year for methylphenidate in the U.S. alone, and another six million are written for various amphetamine compounds such as Adderall.[31] These drugs are useful in decreasing manic behavior in hyperactive children and adults. The mechanism for the paradoxical response in these populations (i.e., why taking a stimulant results in a calming) is not fully understood.[32]

When taking methylphenidate, children who were previously unable to concentrate and had difficulty learning were able to perform at their age-appropriate level. Tolerance and dependence do not develop in children who are taking these medications. A slowing of growth has been observed when children take methylphenidate for long periods. To remedy this, children are given "drug vacations" from their medication on weekends and/or over the summer when they are not in school. Usually this break allows children to catch up on their growth if it has been slowed due to the medication.

Methylphenidate and amphetamine can be drugs of abuse. They can be dissolved and injected for a rapid effect (drug "rush"). When used in this manner, they have effects like cocaine, but milder. A tolerance develops if they are used frequently in this way, and withdrawal symptoms will occur after one has become physically dependent.[2]

Atomoxetine

The drug atomoxetine/Strattera is the only FDA-approved treatment for adult ADHD. It is not been classified as a stimulant. For this reason, it is not considered by the DEA to be a controlled substance, so more doctors are willing to prescribe it. A major advantage of this drug is that it only needs to be taken once in the morning, and its effect lasts until evening without causing insomnia. A 13-item, parent-rated diary was developed by the manufacturer to assess efficacy of the drug on their children during the early morning and in the evening. The symptoms evaluated included:

- oppositionality
- hyperactivity/impulsivity
- inattentiveness/distractibility
- inability to concentrate on structured tasks

Atomoxetine was found to be effective in treating these symptoms.[33] There are indications that a reduction in the dose of atomoxetine may be necessary for patients with impaired liver functions.[34] Now that the drug is on the market and is being used much more widely, additional adverse effects may emerge.

Buspirone

Although it was developed as an antianxiety medication and is not considered a stimulant, buspirone/BuSpar has been found to be as effective as methylphenidate in reducing the symptoms of ADHD, with minimal adverse effects. Some children taking buspirone experienced dizziness during the first week of treatment.[35]

Caffeine & ADHD

Caffeine has been shown to have the effect of improving functioning and reducing levels of hyperactivity in children with ADHD. Although traditional treatments with methylphenidate and amphetamines outperform caffeine in improving functioning, caffeine outperforms the control groups getting no treatment. Some improvements are:

- better relationships with parents and teachers
- reduced aggression   • reduced impulsiveness
- reduced hyperactivity • improved executive functioning[34]

This evidence indicates that caffeine is helpful for children with ADHD and may be valuable as an alternative to the more potent stimulants.[36] Opinions differ on whether caffeine use in children is harmful. No long-term studies have been done to assess its effects on physical and psychological functioning in children. Most children respond to caffeine in the same way as adults. There is a stimulating effect, observed as nervousness, and response time is shortened.[36]

Caffeine may be a tolerable option for parents who are opposed to the use of other stimulants due to fear of long-term adverse effects on their children.

Stimulants for Treatment of Depression

The amphetamines and methylphenidate may be appropriate for short-term use to treat depression, but due to fears of their addictive potential, they are not frequently prescribed.[37] Stimulants can be useful for treating depression when apathy and lack of motivation are present. These drugs can help to get someone launched on a regime of exercise and constructive activities that support the maintenance of an elevated mood. Their virtue is that these drugs act immediately, while most antidepressants take several weeks to reach their maximal effect. Immediacy can be critical if a patient is suicidal. It is the immediacy of response which also makes stimulants potential drugs of abuse. People who have no history of addiction usually do not become addicted when taking these drugs for therapeutic purposes.[38]

Direct Relevance to Psychotherapy

It is very important to be aware that a paranoid psychosis may result from long-term use of stimulant drugs (particularly with amphetamines or cocaine). This drug-related condition may be clinically indistinguishable from the paranoid psychosis seen with schizophrenia or during a manic episode. The symptoms include:

- hostility
- paranoia
- delusions
- aggressiveness
- disorganized thought patterns
- hallucinations (usually auditory)

These psychotic symptoms occur most often when there is a sudden increase in dosage, or in chronic users of amphetamines who are taking more than 100 mg/day. The treatment of choice for this drug-induced psychosis is to stop the stimulant use and begin a course of antipsychotic medication. Recovery from a drug-induced psychosis is not always immediate; it may take days or weeks to clear. In some cases, the psychosis may last for years and require continuing the antipsychotic medication. Autopsy results show that heavy amphetamine use can cause permanent brain damage.[39]

Each therapist's family history and personal experiences with smoking and the diseases it causes will strongly influence his or her feelings about tobacco and its associated ills. There is no denying that tobacco use is a health hazard. Consumption of nicotine, like any other addictive drug or unhealthy habit, deserves exploration in therapy. For clients who want to stop, cognitive and behavioral interventions have proven to be most effective for changing habits. The psychotherapist can discuss with the client whether a medication like bupropion or naltrexone might be desired in addition to psychotherapy. Studies demonstrate that using a nicotine patch in conjunction with bupropion while continuing in therapy leads to significantly higher long-term rates of cessation than the use of either of these alone.[26]

References for Chapter 6

1. Stahl, S. M. (1999). Awakening to the psychopharmacology of sleep and arousal: Novel neurotransmitters and wake-promoting drugs. *J. Clinical Psychiatry*, 63(4), 339–402.
2. Chiang, W. K., MD & Goldfrank, L. R., MD. (1990). Substance withdrawal. *Emergency Medicine Clinics of North America,* Aug., 8(3), 613–614.
3. Methamphetamine information: History of methamphetamine. Retrieved Dec. 7, 2003, from
   http://www.narconon.org/druginfo/methamphetamine_hist.html
4. Johnson, B. A. (2000). Ondansetron for reduction of drinking among biologically predisposed alcoholic patients. *JAMA,* 284(8), 36.
5. Krol, C. (2003). The coca plant. Retrieved Dec. 7, 2003 from
   http://www.siu.edu/~ebl/leaflets/coca2.htm
6. Gerasimov, M. R., Schiffer, W. K., Brodie, J. D., Lennon, I. C., Taylor, S. J. & Dewey, S. L. (2000). gamma-Aminobutyric acid mimetic drugs differentially inhibit the dopaminergic response to cocaine. *Eur. J. Pharmacol.,* 395(2), 129–135.
7. Petrakis, I. L., Carrol, K. M., Nich, C., Gordon, L. T., McCance-Katz, E. F., Frankforter, T. & Rounsaville, B. J. (2000). Disulfiram treatment for cocaine dependence in methadone-maintained opioid addicts. *Addiction,* 95(2), 219–228.
8. Raby, W. N. & Coomaraswamy, S. (2004). Gabapentin reduces cocaine use among addicts from a community clinic sample. *J. Clin. Psychiatry,* 65(1), 84–86.
9. Dackis, C. A., Kampman, K. M., Pettinati, H. & O'brien, C. B. (2003). Effect of modafinil on cocaine abstinence and treatment retention in cocaine dependence: Preliminary results from open-label study. American Psychiatric Assn. 156th Annual Meeting; May, 2003; San Francisco, CA. Abstract S&CR1-4.
10. Sussman, E. (1997). Cocaine vaccine is almost ready for the market. *Psychopharmacology Update,* 8(2), 1, 7.
11. Foxhall, K. (2001). Preventing Relapse. *Monitor on Psychology,* June 46–47.
12. Carpenter, S. (2001). Mixing medication and psychosocial therapy for alcoholism. *Monitor on Psychology,* June, 36–37.
13. Golender, L. & Beuquet. (2003). History of Tea: Botanics. Retrieved Dec. 7, 2003 from http://www.geocities.com/lgol27/HistoryTeaBotanics.htm
14. The coffee plant: Tree to cup/Harvesting. Retrieved Dec. 7, 2003 from

http://www.realcoffee.co.uk/Article.asp?Cat=TreeToCup&Page=1

15. Hughes, J. R., Higgins, S. T., Bickel, W. K., Hunt, W. K., Fenwick, J. W., Gulliver, S. B. & Mireault, G. C. (1991). Caffeine self-administration, withdrawal, and adverse effects among coffee drinkers. *Archives of General Psychiatry*, 48, 611–617.

16. Charney, G. S.; Henninger, G. R. & Jatlow, P. I. (1985). Increased anxiogenic effects of caffeine in panic disorders. *Archives of General Psychiatry*, 42, 233–243.

17. Bruce, M. & Lader, M. (1989). Caffeine abstention in the management of anxiety disorders *Psychological Medicine*, 19, 221–214.

18. Borio, G. (2003). The history of tobacco: Part 1. Retrieved Dec. 7, 2003 from http://www.historian.org/bysubject/tobacco1.htm

19. Wetter, D. E., Fiore, M. C., Gritz, E. R., Lando, H. A., Stitzer, M. L., Hasselblad, V. & Baker, T. B. (1998). The agency for health care policy and research, smoking cessation clinical practice guideline, findings and implications for psychologists. *American Psychologist*, 53(6), 657–669.

20. *Morbidity and Mortality Weekly Report.* (1997). 46(20), 444–451.

21. Parrott, A. C. (1999). Does cigarette smoking cause stress? *American Psychologist*, 54(10), 817–820.

22. Breslau, N., Kilbey, M. & Andreski, P. (1991). Nicotine dependence, major depression and anxiety in young adults. *Arch. Gen. Psychiatry*, 48, 1069–1074.

23. Walton, R., Johnstone, E. & Munafo, M. (2001). Genetic clues to the molecular basis of tobacco addiction and progress towards personalized therapy. *Trends Mol. Med.*, 7(2), 70–76.

24. Leistikow, B. N., MD, MS, Martin, D., Jacobs, J., MD, MPH, & Sherman, C., PHD. (1996). A meta-analysis of the prospective association between smoking and suicide. *J. Addictive Diseases*, 15, 141.

25. McChargue, D. E., PHD., Gulliver, S. B., PHD. & Hitsman, B., PHD. (2003). Applying a stepped-care reduction approach to smokers with schizophrenia. *Psychiatric Times*, Sept., 78.

26. Jorenby, G. B., Leischow, S. J., Nides, M. A., Rennard, S. I., Johnston, J. A., Huges, A. R., Smith, S. S., Muramoto, M. L., Daughton, D. M., Doan, K., Fiore, M. C. & Baker, T. B. (1999). A control trial of sustained-release bupropion, a nicotine patch, or both for smoking cessation. *New England Journal of Medicine*, 340, 685–691.

27. Ahmadi J., Ashkani H., Ahmadi M. & Ahmadi N. (2003). Twenty-four week maintenance treatment of cigarette smoking with nicotine gum, clonidine and naltrexone. *J. Subst. Abuse Treat.* 24(3), 251–255.

28. Dewey, S. L., Brodie, J. D., Gerasimov, M., Horan, B., Gardner, E. L. & Ashby, C. R. (1999). A pharmacologic strategy for the treatment of nicotine addiction. *Synapse,* 31(1), 76–86.

29. Wender, E. H. (2002). Attention-deficit/hyperactivity disorder: Is it common? Is it overtreated? *Arch. Pediatr. Adolesc. Med.*, 156, 209–210.

30. History of methylphenidate. Retrieved Dec. 7, 2003 from http://www.repsych.ac.uk/traindev/epd/adhd/drug/mpd1.htm

31. DEA Congressional Testimony, Caucus on International Narcotics Control, July 25, 2000, Fiano, R. A. US Dept. of Justice, Drug Enforcement Administration.

32. Gainetdinov, R. R., Wetsel, W. C., Jones, S. R., Levin, E. D., Jaber, M. & Caron, M. G. R. (1999). Role of serotonin in the paradoxical calming effect of psychostimulants on hyperactivity. *Science*, 283(5400), 397–401.

33. Michaelson, D., Adler, L., Spencer, T., Reimherr, F. W., West, S. A., Allen, A. J., Wernicke, J., Dietrich, A. & Milton, D. (2003). Atomoxetine in adults with ADHD: Two randomized, placebo-controlled studies. *Biol. Psychiatry*, 53(2), 112–20.

34. Chalon, S. A. (2003). Hepatic impairment with atomoxetine. *Clin. Pharmacol. Ther.*, 73, 178–191.

35. Malhotra, S. & Santosh, P. J. (1998). An open clinical trial of buspirone in children with attention-deficit/hyperactivity disorder. *J. Am. Acad. Child Adolesc. Psychiatry*, 37, 364–371.

36. O'Connor, E. (2001). A slip into dangerous territory. *Monitor on Psychology*, June, 60–62.

37. Wagner, J. G., Rabkin, J. G. & Rabkin, R. (1997). Dextroamphetamine as a treatment for depression and low energy in AIDS patients: A pilot study. *Psychosomatic Research,* April, 42(4), 407–411.

38. Satel, S. L. & Nelson, J. C. (1989). No reports of addiction using stimulants under medical supervision. *J. Clin. Psychiatry*, July 50(7), 241–249.

39. Eisch, A. J., Schmued, L. C. & Marshall, J. F. (1998). Characterizing cortical neuron injury with fluro-jade labeling after a neurotoxic regimen of methamphetamine. *Synapse*, 3, 329.

Chapter 7

Treatment of Psychotic Disorders

Since the 1940's, many drugs and other procedures, including insulin shock and ECT, have been used to treat psychosis. Psychosis can be broadly defined as the loss of contact with reality (the presence of hallucinations and delusions). Although individual patients may respond to one drug or another, to date it has not been demonstrated that any one drug is more effective overall than any other. One patient may respond well

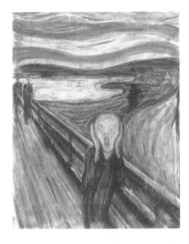

to a particular antipsychotic medication, but not to another, while a second patient, with a similar history and symptoms, may respond very differently. There is no reliable method for predicting how any individual will react to any particular antipsychotic drug.

Psychoactive drugs are often selected based on their side-effect profile. For example, different antipsychotic drugs cause different levels of sedation, an important factor in determining which to use. The psychiatrist, aware of these variables, evaluates which drug has the best chance of working and will have the fewest, and least dangerous, adverse effects for each individual patient.

Schizophrenia

About 1% of the population suffers from schizophrenia.[1] There is strong evidence that this disease has a genetic component. Children of one schizophrenic parent have a 13% chance of becoming schizophrenic whether or not the child has been raised with the schizophrenic parent. There is a 48% concordance rate in monozygotic (identical) twins and a 13% rate in dizygotic (fraternal) twins. These statistics suggest the influence of both genetic and environmental factors in the occurrence of schizophrenia.[1]

Positive & negative symptoms of schizophrenia

The symptoms of schizophrenia are characterized as either positive or negative. These terms do not indicate whether a symptom is "good" or "bad." Positive symptoms refer to things like hallucinations, hearing voices, and delusions that are present only in the patient's mind, whereas negative symptoms refer to the absence of some quality (e.g., turning inward, anhedonia, apathy, social withdrawal). New antipsychotic drugs are constantly being developed in the hopes that they will have fewer adverse effects and increased efficacy, in particular with regard to negative symptoms.[2]

Antipsychotic Medications

The drugs used to treat psychotic symptoms have been called by many different names: major tranquilizers, phenothiazine tranquilizers, neuroleptics, and antipsychotic medications. To avoid confusion, the term "antipsychotic" will be used in this book to refer to all the drugs in this class. These will be categorized as: first generation antipsychotics (FGAs); second generation antipsychotics (SGAs); and a group of antipsychotic drugs called dopamine system stabilizers (DSSs) which have recently become available.

As the name antipsychotic indicates, this class of drugs is used for the treatment of psychoses, usually for the psychotic symptoms present in schizophrenia. They are also used to treat psychotic symptoms that may occur during a depression or during a manic episode. When prescribed to treat a psychotic episode that is part of a depression or a bipolar disorder, they are taken on a short-term basis (four to five months), whereas with a diagnosis of schizophrenia they are generally taken over much longer periods, often for years.

Time-course for antipsychotic medications

When antipsychotic medication is started, there may be a period (sometimes as long as 12 weeks) of gradual improvement in psychotic symptoms.[3] During this time, psychotherapy can consist of dealing with the practicalities of life and nurturing the development of a therapeutic alliance. A client who has psychotic symptoms often needs assistance and support getting along in the world on a day-to-day basis, at work or school, learning to deal with family, and developing social skills. The therapist can help the client learn how to make simple decisions such as what type of milk to buy, as well as how to master complex tasks, like applying for a job, and to develop ways to become more self-sufficient in general.

Optimal treatment for a client on medication requires a collaborative relationship between psychotherapist and psychiatrist. The psychotherapist sees the patient much more frequently, and may be the first to notice a disturbing adverse effect of a medication. If this occurs, a consultation with the psychiatrist is necessary to discuss the symptoms observed. The psychiatrist will then be the one to evaluate whether or not a serious condition is developing. Ongoing monitoring of the client by the therapist is important since some serious adverse effects (such as *tardive dyskinesia*) can emerge even after the patient has been on medication for a long period of time, sometimes years.[3]

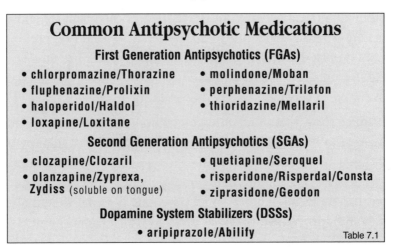

Common Antipsychotic Medications

First Generation Antipsychotics (FGAs)

- chlorpromazine/Thorazine
- fluphenazine/Prolixin
- haloperidol/Haldol
- loxapine/Loxitane
- molindone/Moban
- perphenazine/Trilafon
- thioridazine/Mellaril

Second Generation Antipsychotics (SGAs)

- clozapine/Clozaril
- olanzapine/Zyprexa, Zydiss (soluble on tongue)
- quetiapine/Seroquel
- risperidone/Risperdal/Consta
- ziprasidone/Geodon

Dopamine System Stabilizers (DSSs)

- aripiprazole/Abilify

Table 7.1

Effects of Antipsychotic Medications

There is evidence that schizophrenia is primarily due to a disturbance in the DA systems in the CNS. It is believed that some parts of the brain have too little DA, and other parts have too much. Antipsychotic medications attempt to correct these imbalances.[4]

Usually the first effect seen is sedation; the patient becomes calmer in several hours. This sedation is particularly valuable for treating manic patients, or for those who have violent, self-destructive, or suicidal delusions. Patients develop a tolerance to this effect in about two weeks. After several weeks, patients report that their delusions, disordered thinking, and hallucinations either have disappeared, decreased, or that they are no longer bothered by them.

Many patients who are having a first psychotic episode and are put on medication will have a full remission of the hallucinations or delusions. If kept on medication, the possibility of a relapse is greatly reduced but not eliminated.[3] Relapse rate for patients maintained on antipsychotic medication is 15% to 30% in the first year, whereas patients not kept on medication have a relapse rate of 50% to 70%. When medication is discontinued, at least 40% of patients have a relapse within six months.[3]

No tolerance develops to the antipsychotic effect of these drugs and they do not cause euphoria, so there is no potential for abuse or addiction. There is evidence to suggest that repeated or prolonged psychotic episodes will gradually make the schizophrenic disorder worse. Patients become discouraged and more socially isolated, and recovery often takes longer and becomes more difficult.[3]

Studies show that psychotherapy without medication is no better than placebo for treating an acute psychosis, and that therapy with medication is no better than medication alone for treating an acute psychotic state. For long-term treatment, therapy and medication are better than medication alone. With psychotic patients, therapy helps most with improvement of social skills and social adjustment.[5]

First Generation Antipsychotics (FGAs)

This group, also called "traditional" or "classical" antipsychotic drugs, has many adverse effects.

EXTRAPYRAMIDAL SYNDROME (EPS)

The most frequently seen adverse effects with FGAs are various movement disorders collectively called extrapyramidal syndrome (EPS). It is believed that EPS occurs when 78% of the DA receptors in the CNS are occupied with an antipsychotic medication.[5] Onset of EPS is clearly a dose-related effect of FGAs, and occurs in at least 10% of all patients on FGAs. Some EPS symptoms, particularly the presence of a tremor, resemble Parkinson's disease. Symptoms of EPS can last for several months. These symptoms are low with the SGAs, and occur very infrequently with clozapine/Clozaril.[5]

Treatment of EPS with anticholinergic drugs

There has always been a question as to the advisability of whether drugs to prevent EPS should be given at the start of FGA medication, or whether to wait for EPS to occur and then start treatment. Some patients become very frightened, and refuse to continue taking antipsychotic medication if extrapyramidal symptoms occur. For this reason, many physicians will prescribe trihexyphenidyl/Artane or benztropine/Cogentin as a preventive measure before any symptoms of EPS appear. Others argue that because not all patients get EPS many do not need these extra medications since these drugs also have adverse effects which must be weighed against their potential benefits. The anticholinergic drugs most frequently used to treat EPS are benztropine and trihexyphenidyl.[5]

The anticholinergic drugs cause a decrease in the amount of ACh available to the neurons; this leads to decreased movement and a reversal of the EPS. These drugs also decrease anxiety and depression and may improve the negative symptoms of schizophrenia. Their adverse effects are:

- dry mouth • nausea
- dizziness • blurred near vision

The elderly, due to their already decreased levels of ACh, may have more severe complications, such as urinary retention and delirium.[5]

Treatment of EPS with amantadine/Symmetrel

The antiviral drug amantadine increases DA release, which leads to a decrease in EPS. Adverse effects of amantadine include:

- dizziness • insomnia
- seizures   • psychotic symptoms[5]

TARDIVE DYSKINESIA (TD)

TD is a serious adverse effect caused by many FGAs. TD can appear at any time from three months to ten years after beginning medication. Frequently seen symptoms are:

- hand clenching
- finger movements such as choreiform (dance-like) movements
- oral and facial movements such as torticolis (tightening of neck and face muscles)[6]

The rate of occurrence of TD in patients on FGA medications is 3% to 4% per year for the first five years. TD occurs most often in patients who have been maintained for many years on high doses of traditional antipsychotic medications. As many as 50% of patients who were treated with these medications on a chronic basis developed TD.[7]

TD is reversible in more than 30% of patients if the antipsychotic medication is discontinued. For the rest, the TD does not remit even when medication is discontinued. TD does not respond to anticholinergic medication, even though this is the usual treatment for movement disorders like EPS. Prolonged treatment with anticholinergic drugs may increase the chance of later development TD.[6]

Etiology of TD

The specific cause of TD is not yet known. One theory is that TD is due to hypersensitivity or over-proliferation of DA receptors, caused by the body's effort to maintain a state of homeostasis, by growing new receptors to compensate for those blocked by medication. Symptoms of TD can be temporarily diminished by increasing the dosage of antipsychotic medication, but over time this remedy will intensify symptoms. As scientific understanding of the complexity of the CNS and the various neurotransmitter and neuromodulator systems increases, so does the complexity of the various theories about the underlying mechanisms for TD.[7]

Treatment of TD

Reserpine, lithium, vitamin E, or BZs sometimes are effective in alleviating TD. Vitamin E and ondansetron/Zofran, a 5-HT antagonist, may prove to be an effective treatment for both TD and psychotic symptoms.[8] Reserpine depletes NE, DA, and 5-HT stores; when taken for two to four days, it can relieve symptoms of TD, but may also cause a serious depression.[7] Most psychiatrists proceed by taking the patient off the antipsychotic medication and changing the medication to clozapine or to one of the newer SGAs that have a lower incidence of TD. The newer drugs are believed to have their site of action more in the limbic system and on 5-HT, and less on DA striatal neurons; for this reason they are less likely to cause movement disorders.[2] As of this writing, there is no definitive, successful treatment for TD.

Effects of antipsychotic medications on the hypothalamus

Antipsychotic drugs have specific effects on the hypothalamus. Frequently seen are:

- decreased appetite • impotence in men
- infertility in women (decreased ovulation)
- decreased libido (decreased production of testosterone)
- decreased adaptability to external temperature changes[5]

Antipsychotic drugs cause little or no respiratory depression. They do cause a decrease in seizure threshold, making the possibility of a seizure more likely. They can also cause:

- lactation   • weight gain
- impairment in liver function leading to jaundice
- formation of pigment deposits on the retina leading to impaired vision [5]

NEUROLEPTIC MALIGNANT SYNDROME (NMS)

Neuroleptic malignant syndrome is a serious, sometimes fatal disorder caused by antipsychotic medications. Symptoms include:

- sweating   • altered mental state
- renal (kidney) failure   • high fever (up to 107°F)
- elevated white blood cell count
- increased pulse and respiration rate
- severe Parkinsonian muscle rigidity (can make walking or talking difficult or impossible) [9]

NMS can occur when starting on medication or when the patient has already been stabilized on it. It can appear in someone who in the past took antipsychotic medication without problems and then, when restarted on the same medication, develops NMS. The syndrome develops quickly, over a period of 24 to 72 hours. NMS can persist from 10 to 14 days with shorter-acting preparations, or for as long as four weeks with the long-acting, depot preparations.

Amantadine, bromocriptine, and L-dopa are sometimes helpful in alleviating NMS; this is probably due to their ability to cause an increase in dopamine activity in the CNS. ECT is also an effective treatment. The usual treatment regimen consists of discontinuing medication, hospitalization, and initiation of life-support measures. Estimates of the rate of occurrence of NMS range from 0.02% to 2.4% for all patients on antipsychotic medications. The fatality rate is high, approximately 20%. [9]

Risk factors for NMS

Psychotherapists who are seeing patients who are taking antipsychotic medications need to know which patients are at the greatest risk of developing NMS. There are some clear indications as to who this will be. About 80% of affected patients are under age 40, and males are affected twice as often as females. There is also a direct correlation between the risk of getting NMS and a history of:

- psychomotor agitation • higher doses of medication
- rapid increase in dose of medication
- high number of intramuscular medication injections [9]

Studies have shown that both the maximum amount of medication, and the total number of doses, were nine times greater in patients with NMS than in the control group of patients who did not get NMS. The mean number of intramuscular injections received was also nine times greater than that of the control group. [9]

Intramuscular administration causes higher peak levels of the drug in the blood stream leading to an abrupt blockade of DA in the CNS. The rapid blockage of DA may not allow enough time for they body's compensatory mechanisms that maintain homeostasis of life-support functions controlled in the CNS to take effect. [9]

The usual sequence of events for patients who develop NMS is this: A young male comes to an Emergency Room with symptoms of agitation and psychosis; he is given an injection of antipsychotic medication to calm him rapidly and to treat the psychotic symptoms. It is this rapid administration of a high dose of antipsychotic medication which seems to precipitate NMS. If you are treating patients at a high risk for NMS, be sure to inform them of their risk. If any symptoms of NMS appear, the patient needs to be hospitalized and treated as soon as possible. [9]

Depot preparations

In the 1960's some long-acting, injectable forms of antipsychotic medications called "depot" preparations were developed with the hope of improving patient compliance and thus reducing the rate of relapse and rehospitalization. In these long-acting preparations, the active drug is suspended in an inactive carrier and is administered via subcutaneous or intramuscular injection. The carrier causes the drug to be absorbed slowly, so the medication only needs to be administered every one or two weeks. The major problem is that there is no way to quickly remove the drug from the body if adverse effects do occur. As a safeguard, patients are put on depot preparations only after a trial with a shorter-acting form of the same drug. There is no increased risk of NMS or TD with depot preparations.[10]

Because the drug does not pass through the digestive tract to get into the bloodstream, stable blood-levels are easier to maintain, and the dose can be lower than when taken orally. Many people dislike or are fearful of injections, so depot preparations are not widely used. They are used primarily with patients who have compliance problems with oral medications or for people who don't like the idea of taking pills every day.[10]

Drug manufacturers are currently at work developing various long-acting preparations of the SGAs. One preparation of risperidone/Consta, designed to be injected and effective for two weeks, is now approved and available for use in the United States.

Second Generation Antipsychotics (SGAs)

Manufacturers are continually developing new antipsychotic drugs with the hope of finding compounds that are effective in the treatment of the symptoms of schizophrenia and do not cause TD or other serious adverse effects. The newer drugs are called "second generation antipsychotics" (SGAs); this category includes the antipsychotics formerly called "atypical" or "novel." These agents act as antagonists at 5-HT receptors as well as at DA receptors. SGAs include: clozapine, olanzapine, quetiapine, risperidone, and ziprasidone.

Clozapine (the prototype SGA)

Often considered in a class by itself, clozapine/Clozaril was the first of this group of drugs to be developed and is the prototype for those that followed. Introduced into clinical practice in Europe in 1975, it is used to treat psychoses, *Tourette's syndrome* (a disorder with symptoms of verbal and motor tics), and for the psychotic symptoms that are sometimes induced by the drug L-dopa, which is used to treat Parkinson's disease. Clozapine is unique in that it does not cause TD,[13] and for this reason it has been of great interest to researchers and drug companies as well as to patients, and the families of patients, who need to take antipsychotic medication.

Adverse effects of clozapine

Clozapine produces minimal EPS and can even be used as a treatment for TD.[11] The reason it is not the first drug of choice for psychotic symptoms is that it can cause a serious, potentially life-threatening disorder called agranulocytosis (a blood disorder with a high fatality rate). The incidence of agranulocytosis is approximately 1% to 2% for patients taking clozapine, a rate ten times higher than occurs with any other antipsychotic drug. The agranulocytosis can be reversed if clozapine treatment is stopped within two weeks of development of the disorder.[5] When on clozapine, the patient's blood must be monitored on a weekly basis for the first six months. If there are no signs of agranulocytosis, the frequency of the monitoring can be reduced to once every two weeks. The manufacturer will not supply clozapine if the monitoring is not done. Monitoring is required for as long as clozapine is taken.

Rather than a toxic effect, agranulocytosis seems to be an autoimmune response of the bone marrow to clozapine.[5] The peak for its occurrence is in the first four months of treatment, although cases throughout the first year have been reported. Because of the life-threatening nature of this adverse effect, clozapine is usually only given when patients have not responded to other antipsychotic medications. Thirty percent of patients who do not respond to other antipsychotic drugs will respond to clozapine, although the first signs of improvement may not be seen for four to six months.[12]

Other possible adverse effects of clozapine are:

- seizures
- sedation
- weight gain

- hypotension
- excessive salivation
- tachycardia (rapid heartbeat)[5]

For some patients, clozapine causes more of a dramatic improvement in social functioning than in psychotic symptoms.[2] Improvement in social functioning is a rare and desirable quality sought after by manufacturers, doctors, and patients. Unfortunately, agranulocytosis can be life-threatening, and many patients refuse the frequent blood draws. Some patients who have a very good response to clozapine will not tolerate the blood tests and therefore cannot continue taking it.

Other SGAs

Some antipsychotic medications have been developed to replicate clozapine's positive effects and eliminate its adverse effects. Among these are the newer drugs olanzapine/Zyprexa, risperidone/Risperdal, quetiapine/Seroquel, and ziprasidone/Geodon. None of these is as effective as clozapine for people who have not responded to other antipsychotic drugs. They all cause a lower rate of EPS and TD than the FGAs, and they all claim to improve negative symptoms, but clozapine remains unique in its ability to prevent TD. Ziprasidone may cause cognitive improvement when compared with other antipsychotic drugs.[13] There is evidence that olanzapine may be useful in the treatment of borderline personality disorder.[14]

Other adverse effects of SGAs

There is strong evidence that taking many of the SGAs will lead to impaired glucose metabolism. This impairment leads to weight gain and diabetes.[15] When on these medications patients need additional counseling about nutrition, exercise, hyperglycemia, and diabetes. The effect on glucose tolerance usually abates when the drug is stopped. Most of the SGAs cause significant weight gain. At the end of a five-year study of patients treated with clozapine, approximately 30% were diagnosed with Type II diabetes. Diabetes was reported in 33% of patients taking olanzapine. No significant changes in weight have been attributed to ziprasidone. It is recommended that patients on SGAs be monitored for diabetes with a blood test every six months. [12, 15-17]

There is some evidence that nizatidine/Axid (used to treat ulcers) may decrease the amount of weight gained by patients taking olanzapine (an SGA) by 50%. There also has been some success using metformin (oral insulin used to treat Type II diabetes) for weight loss with children taking SGAs.[18, 19]

Dopamine System Stabilizers (DSSs)

A new group of antipsychotic drugs, dopamine system stabilizers (DSSs), is now available. The first drug in this group, aripiprazole/Abilify is said to be useful for controlling both the positive and negative symptoms of schizophrenia. It seems to have fewer adverse effects than other antipsychotic medications. Most common adverse effects of aripiprazole are:

- nausea
- insomnia
- anxiety
- headache
- constipation [20, 21]

The manufacturer claims that its use will not lead to the weight gain and the development of diabetes seen with most SGAs.

Sarcosine: an Amino Acid for Schizophrenia

Taking sarcosine, a naturally occurring amino acid, can lead to improvement of symptoms of schizophrenia. Sarcosine is believed to work by blocking glycine reuptake; this leads to an activation of the NMDA receptor. Drugs that target this mechanism have been moderately successful in treating some symptoms of schizophrenia.[22]

Dehydroepiandrosterone (DHEA) for Negative Symptoms of Schizophrenia

There has been little success to date using medications to treat the negative symptoms of schizophrenia such as anhedonia, flat affect, and social isolation. One recent study has shown that administering DHEA to patients along with other antipsychotic medication led to a significant reduction in negative symptoms.[23]

An Alternative Treatment for Psychosis

Some valiant attempts have been made to treat psychotic patients in an environment where patients were not medicated and where there was round-the-clock care. One of these was Diabasis House, started in San Francisco in 1974 by John Perry. The design of our current health-care system does not support this type of intensive treatment, since a large number of personnel is necessary to support patients as they go through psychotic episodes.[24] Since treatment settings like Diabasis House are very rare, therapists have few opportunities to explore the validity of these modes of treatment. For these reasons, use of antipsychotic medication is the primary method currently used to treat positive psychotic symptoms.

Direct Relevance to Psychotherapy

Most therapists agree it is difficult to do effective psychotherapy with a person who is delusional. It is important to first get the positive symptoms under control, usually with medication, and then proceed with psychotherapy to work on the negative symptoms.

To understand how medications are most appropriately used in the treatment of schizophrenia, it is helpful to examine the symptoms in the categories of "positive," more overt symptoms, and "negative," less obvious, more asocial features. Negative symptoms usually increase over time, and positive symptoms usually decrease. Each person may experience different proportions of positive and negative symptoms throughout the course of the disease; some individuals may experience more of one type of symptom than the other. Most antipsychotic medications treat the positive symptoms of schizophrenia, but do not have much influence on the negative symptoms. Psychotherapy can greatly impact negative symptoms, but usually does not have much influence on positive symptoms. Therefore, the combination of medication and psychotherapy is usually necessary in order to provide optimal treatment for patients with psychotic disorders.

References for Chapter 7

1. Gottesman, I. I. (2001). Psychopathology through a life span-genetic perspective. *American Psychologist,* November, 867–878.
2. Meltzer, H. Y. (1992). Dimensions of outcome with clozapine, *British J. of Psychiatry,* 160(suppl. 17), 46–53.
3. Wyatt, R. J. (1991). Neuroleptics and the natural course of schizophrenia. *Schizophrenia Bulletin,* 7(2), 325–351.
4. Singh, A. N., Barlas, C., Singh, S., Franks, P. & Mishra, R. K. (1996). A neurochemical basis for the antipsychotic activity of loxapine: Interactions with dopamine D1, D2, D4 and serotonin 5-HT2 receptor subtypes. *J. Psychiatry Neurosci.,* 21(1), 29–35.
5. *The Merck manual of diagnosis and therapy.* (2001). (17th ed.). Rahway, NJ: Merck Sharp & Dohme Research Laboratories.
6. Lieberman, J., MD. (1989). Dopamine pathophysiology in tardive dyskinesia. *Psychiatric Annals,* 19(6), 35–40.
7. Szymanski, S., DO., Munne, R., MD., Gordon, M. F., MD. & Lieberman, J., MD. (1993). A selective review of recent advances in the management of tardive dyskinesia. *Psychiatric Annals,* 23(4), 41–47.
8. Sirota P., Mosheva T., Shabtay, H., Giladi, N. & Korczyn, A. D. (2000). Use of the selective serotonin 3 receptor antagonist ondansetron in the treatment of neuroleptic-induced tardive dyskinesia. *Am. J. Psychiatry,* 157, 287–289.
9. Viejo, L. F., Morales, V., Punal, J. L. & Sancho, R. A. (2003). Risk factors in neuroleptic malignant syndrome. A case control study. *Acta. Psychiatr. Scand.,* Jan, 107, 45–49.
10. Glazer, W. M., MD & Kane, J. M., MD. (1992). Depot neuroleptic therapy: An underutilized treatment option. *J. Clinical Psychiatry,* 53, 426–433.
11. Meltzer, H. Y. & Luchins, D. J. (1984). Effect of clozapine in serve tardive dyskinesia: A case report. *J. Clin. Psychopharm.,* 4(5), 286–287.
12. Honigfeld, G., Patin, J. & Singer, J. (1984). Clozapine: Antipsychotic activity in

treatment-resistant schizophrenics. *Adv. Ther.,* 1(2), 77–79.

13. Harvey, P. D., Meltzer, H., Simpson, G. M., Potkin, S. G., Loebel, A., Siu, C. & Romano, S. J. (2004). Improvement in cognitive function following a switch to ziprasidone from conventional antipsychotics, olanzapine, or risperidone in outpatients with schizophrenia. *Schizophrenia Research,* 66(2–3), 101–113.

14. Bogenschutz, M. P. & Nurnberg, G. H. (2004). Olanzapine vs. placebo in the treatment of borderline personality disorder. *J. Clinical Psychiatry,* 65(1), 104–109.

15. Goldstein, L. E. & Henderson, D. C. (2000). Atypical antipsychotic agents and diabetes mellitus. *Primary Psychiatry,* 7(5), 65–68.

16. Newcomer, J. W., Haupt, D. W. & Fucetola, R. (2002). Abnormalities in glucose regulation during antipsychotic treatment of schizophrenia. *Arch. Gen. Psychiatry,* 59, 337–345.

17. Sernyak, M. J., Leslie, D. L., Alarcon, R. D., Losonczy, M. F. & Rosenheck, R. (2002). Association of diabetes mellitus with use of atypical neuroleptics in the treatment of schizophrenia. *Am. J. Psychiatry,* 159(4), 561–566.

18. Cavazzoni, P., Tanaka, Y., Roychowdhury, S. M., Breier, A. & Allison, D. B. (2003). Nizatidine for prevention of weight gain with olanzapine: A double-blind placebo-controlled trial. *Eur. Neuropsychopharm.,* Mar., 13(2), 81–85.

19. Hinney, A., Hoch, A., Geller, F., Schafer, H., Siegfried, W. & Goldschmidt, H. (2002). Ghrelin gene: Identification of missense variants and a frameshift mutation in extremely obese children and adolescents and healthy normal weight students. *J. Clin. Endricinol. Metab.,* 87, 2716.

20. Taylor, D. M. (2003). Aripiprazole: A review of its pharmacology and clinical use. *Int. Journal of Clinical Practice,* 57(1), 49–54.

21. Stahl, S. M. (2001). Dopamine system stabilizers, aripiprazole, and the next generation of antipsychotics, Part I: "Goldilocks" actions at dopamine receptors, and Part II: Illustrating their mechanisms of action. *J. Clinical Psychiatry,* 62(11), 841–842 and 62(12), 923–924.

22. Tsai, G., Lane, H. Y., Yang, P., Chong, M. Y. & Lange, N. (2004). Glycine transporter I inhibitor, N-methylglycine (sarcosine), added to antipsychotics for the treatment of schizophrenia. *Biol. Psychiatry,* 55(5), 452–456.

23. Strous, R. D. (2003). DHEA augmentation for negative symptoms of schizophrenia, *Arch. Gen. Psychiatry,* 60, 133–141.

24. Cornwall, M. W. (2002). Alternative treatment of psychosis: A qualitative study of Jungian medication-free treatment at Diabasis. Doctoral dissertation, California Institute of Integral Studies, San Francisco, CA.

Chapter 8

Pain & Treatments of Pain

It is easier to find men who will volunteer to die than to find those who are willing to endure pain with patience.

Julius Caesar

Pain is one of the most common reasons people seek medical care, with headaches alone accounting for 45 million visits to the doctor in America each year. This number reminds us that many people take over-the-counter or prescription pain medications that can often cause changes in consciousness, memory, and emotional state.

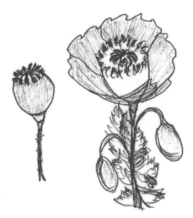

Certain types of pain can only be relieved by potent medications like morphine and other opioid-like

Opium poppy
Papaver somniferum

compounds. Millions of people are forced to rely on these drugs in order to tolerate their pain and be able to have some semblance of a normal life. Pharmacologists have been trying for decades to develop a compound that alleviates deep pain but does not cause physical dependency. As of today, they have not been successful.

SEROTONIN & THE PAIN RESPONSE

Serotonin (5-HT) is one of the many compounds that has a role in the pain response. When 5-HT is depleted, sensitivity to pain increases. The action of morphine on pain requires the presence of 5-HT. Morphine's analgesic effect is blocked when 5-HT is depleted.[1]

Antidepressants are helpful in alleviating certain types of pain, particularly migraine headaches and neurological pain. This is probably due to their effect on 5-HT levels. In the past, these types of pain could only be treated successfully with medications that could cause physical dependence. Taken in low doses, amitriptyline (a TCA which affects NE and 5-HT) is used to decrease the pain caused by arthritic diseases, and has been found to be useful in the treatment of fibromyalgia (a painful rheumatic condition).[2]

Hierarchy of Treatment for Pain

There is a hierarchy in the treatment of pain based upon the side effects and addictive potential of the drugs used. Non-opioid drugs have what is called an "analgesic ceiling," the dose above which no further relief (analgesic effect) can be obtained. Opioids are used when pain cannot be adequately controlled using other treatments. There is no analgesic ceiling with opioids. The dose can be increased until pain is relieved or until side effects become intolerable. Because of variations in drug absorption, metabolism, and each individual's experience of pain, there is no standard opioid dose.[3,4] Most doctors are reluctant to prescribe opioids due to the sedating side effects and addictive potential.[5]

ASPIRIN, NSAIDs, & COX-2 INHIBITORS

When someone is suffering from mild pain, the first drugs usually tried are aspirin and other over-the-counter preparations (e.g., Anacin, Excedrin) or one of the nonsteroidal anti-inflammatory agents (NSAIDs) like ibuprofen/Motrin or naproxen/Aleve, which are useful for treating pain resulting from inflammation. For most people, there are few adverse effects. These may include:

- increased clotting time
- gastric disturbances
- bleeding ulcers or severe irritation of the stomach[6,7]

Warning: These must be taken with food or a full glass of water to avoid the stomach irritation.

Because of their anticoagulant properties, these drugs should not be taken if there is heavy menstrual bleeding or within three weeks of a surgical procedure. The cyclooxygenase-2 (COX-2) inhibitors such as celecoxib/Celebrex (currently available only by prescription) were developed to reduce the risk of stomach irritation caused by aspirin and the NSAIDs.[7]

CORTICOSTEROIDS

Corticosteroids (e.g., prednisone, cortisone) act as anti-inflammatory agents and are utilized in situations where the milder NSAIDs are not adequate. They are often administered by injection directly at the site of the pain for arthritic ailments, such as back pain and bursitis. The most severe adverse effect of these drugs is that, if used frequently in this manner, they eventually destroy bone.[8] If taken long-term, they depress the immune system. Corticosteroids may cause specific psychological symptoms, usually manic episodes with psychotic features. Psychoactive medication may be required to treat these symptoms.

TRANSCUTANEOUS ELECTRICAL NERVE STIMULATION (TENS)

TENS is the administration of an electrical pulse directly to the site of the pain. The pulse is generated by a portable, battery-operated device, worn and controlled by the patient, who self-regulates the pulse as needed. TENS is often used for chronic pain (particularly back pain) when the pain is not very severe and the patient does not want to be constantly taking medication or have the adverse effects of drugs.[9]

ANTIDEPRESSANTS, ANTICONVULSANTS & OTHER DRUGS

Other psychopharmacologic agents are used to treat pain when the above treatments prove inadequate. Many in the following list are discussed in detail elsewhere in this book.

- Anticonvulsant agents (e.g., gabapentin) are useful for neuropathic pain and migraine prophylaxis.[10]

- BZs (e.g., diazepam) are useful for muscle spasm relaxation and restless leg syndrome.
- The herbal agents (e.g., arnica, calendula) are useful for skin injuries and muscle pain.
- Lithium and topiramate are useful for cluster headaches.
- NMDA receptor blockers (e.g., Ketamine, methadone) are useful for *post-herpetic neuralgia.* [11]
- Stimulants (e.g., amphetamines) are used in combination with opioid narcotic agents.[12, 13]
- Topical agents (e.g., capsicum, lidocaine) are useful for arthritic pain.
- TCAs (e.g., amitriptyline) are useful for migraine headaches and fibromyalgia.[14]

OPIUM & OTHER NARCOTIC DRUGS

Opium is the finger of God. It smites, and it heals. It is the gift of heaven when it stills the agonies of death from cancer.
Harry Anslinger, Commissioner
Federal Bureau of Narcotics, 1930–1962

The class of drugs called opioids derives its name from the opium poppy, *Papaver somniferum,* which is native to the Middle East and has been known since ancient times for its strong narcotic effect. The poppy's seed capsule oozes a milky resin, which when collected and dried, becomes opium. Derivatives include morphine, heroin, and

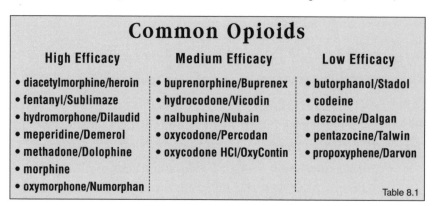

Common Opioids

High Efficacy	Medium Efficacy	Low Efficacy
• diacetylmorphine/heroin	• buprenorphine/Buprenex	• butorphanol/Stadol
• fentanyl/Sublimaze	• hydrocodone/Vicodin	• codeine
• hydromorphone/Dilaudid	• nalbuphine/Nubain	• dezocine/Dalgan
• meperidine/Demerol	• oxycodone/Percodan	• pentazocine/Talwin
• methadone/Dolophine	• oxycodone HCl/OxyContin	• propoxyphene/Darvon
• morphine		
• oxymorphone/Numorphan		Table 8.1

codeine. The opioids as a class contain both natural and synthetic com-pounds that act on the body in ways similar to morphine. All of the opioids selectively bind to specific opioid receptors in the CNS.

Opioid receptors in the CNS

Specific endogenous opioid receptors (different types with dif-ferent behavioral effects) have been found in various parts of the brain. Opioids activate inhibitory pathways in the CNS. When these recep-tors are activated, either with an opioid or via TENS, the pain impulse is inhibited and analgesia results. Opioid receptors that appear to mediate deep pain have been identified; this pain is relieved by opi-oid narcotics, but not by other types of pain medications. Specific areas in the spinal cord are involved in the integration of incoming senso-ry information. There is a decrease in painful stimuli transmitted from the spinal cord to the brain if nerve cells in these areas are inhibited. Acupuncture may work to decrease pain through this pathway.[9, 15-17]

The areas of the limbic system that are associated with emotional responses contain the greatest concentrations of opioid receptors. The amygdala, an area of the brain that controls the anger response, is heavily innervated with opioid receptors. Since these pathways are inhibitory, activation could lead to a decrease in sensitivity to painful physical and emotional stimuli.[17]

The treatment of severe or chronic pain presents many difficulties. Opioids and other derivatives of opium are prescribed only when the milder forms of pain medications and TENS have not been adequate to control the pain. All currently-available opioid pain medications have many adverse effects, including:

- constipation
- loss of appetite
- loss of sexual desire
- physical dependence
- pupillary constriction
- clouding of consciousness [18]

Morphine

Morphine, the chief active ingredient of opium, has both sedative and analgesic properties. Its molecular structure resembles the endorphins, which are the main neurotransmitters involved in the control of pain. Morphine exists in the bloodstream in a water-soluble form and therefore cannot pass easily through the blood-brain barrier. Because of its molecular structure, ten times more heroin than morphine is able to pass through the barrier and into the brain.

Tolerance, cross-tolerance, & overdose

Very large doses of any opioid will cause respiratory depression through inhibition of the respiratory center in the brain stem. Some tolerance to respiratory depression develops with opioids, unlike with barbiturates and alcohol, where little, if any, develops. Tolerance to the analgesic, euphoric, sedative, and emetic (induction of vomiting) effects of opioids develops over time. Very little tolerance develops to the antidiarrhea effect or the pupillary constriction. This is why the presence of "pin-point pupils" is diagnostic for opioid intoxication even in long-term users.[19]

Cross-tolerance develops between different opioids, both natural and synthetic, even ones that are chemically quite dissimilar. Cross-tolerance does not develop between opioids and barbiturates, alcohol, or sedative-hypnotic drugs. Ignorance of this lack of cross-tolerance is the main reason for many of the accidental deaths that result from combining these drugs. This combination can depresses the respiratory centers to such an extent as to lead to coma and death.[19]

All opioids are metabolized by the liver and excreted by the kidneys. Tolerance develops due to both an increase in synthesis of liver enzymes and to a decrease in sensitivity at the opioid receptor.[19] A person suffering from liver or kidney disease has an impaired ability to metabolize opioids; this can lead to a drug accumulation that can reach toxic and overdose levels. The risk of drug overdose is increased for anyone who has had hepatitis or any liver or kidney disease.

ADDICTION TO OPIOIDS

Most people become addicted to opioids due to a desire for euphoric feelings and a blunting of pain. Tolerance to the euphoric effect develops after only one week of daily use. When given morphine for medical purposes (usually every six hours for severe pain), patients develop some physical dependence after only two or three days. Addiction is rare after a brief treatment for severe pain, though when the drug is stopped mild withdrawal symptoms will be experienced. Most people do not like the clouding of consciousness caused by narcotics and do not continue taking them once they can tolerate their pain using non-narcotic medications.[8]

Physical dependence will develop when opioids are taken for chronic and severe pain for long periods of time (weeks or months). In these situations, stopping the drug will be difficult and more severe withdrawal symptoms will occur. Medical supervision or in-patient treatment for withdrawal can be helpful, but is not essential. Although the process of opioid withdrawal is extremely uncomfortable and unpleasant, it is not life-threatening.[19]

Agonist & antagonist

An understanding of the terms "agonist" and "antagonist" is very important in comprehending how various drugs are used to treat opioid addiction and withdrawal. (See Appendix D for a detailed discussion.)

Treatment of opioid overdose

The respiratory depression caused by opioid overdose is usually due to not knowing the actual dose of drug taken or one's exact level of tolerance. These circumstances occur frequently when drugs are obtained illegally. Opioid overdose is usually treated in a hospital emergency room with the opioid antagonists naloxone or nalmefene. Since these are shorter-acting than most opioids, a patient who has overdosed needs to be hospitalized and observed for 24 to 48 hours so that the naloxone or nalmefene treatment can be repeated if necessary. If the patient is not monitored, the opioid antagonist may wear off before the opioid does, and respiratory depression may recur.

In conjunction with reversing the respiratory depression, opiate antagonists bring on symptoms of withdrawal. Severity of withdrawal symptoms is dependent upon:

- the type of opiate used
- the individual's degree of tolerance
- the amount of time since the last dose
- the individual's emotional reaction to the withdrawal symptoms [19]

Naloxone

An injectable (parenteral) pure narcotic antagonist, naloxone/Narcan, has no opiate-like effects. Withdrawal symptoms will occur immediately if naloxone is given to someone addicted to opiates. It is used in emergency rooms in cases of overdose when rapid reversal of respiratory depression is necessary to save the person's life. Naloxone is injected intravenously so that it enters the bloodstream immediately and reaches the brain in about five minutes.[19]

Nalmefene

The opioid antagonist nalmefene/Revex T can be injected intravenously, intramuscularly, or subcutaneously (which can be an advantage if there is difficulty finding a vein). It is longer-acting than naloxone, and has about the same half-life as most opiates. For this reason, it is less likely that repeat doses will be needed. Nalmefene has less of an adverse effect on the liver than naloxone, and may be preferable in cases of overdose.

Treatment of addiction

There are many schools of thought on addiction and the various types of therapies for treating it. Some frequently-used therapies are:

- cognitive therapy
- behavior modification
- pharmacological interventions
- various combinations of all of these
- 12-step programs
- psychodynamic therapy

All of the above methods, alone or in combination, are successful for some people. It is important for the psychotherapist to be aware of the available options and to be able to choose, with the client, the method or methods that might work best. Medications to ease the withdrawal symptoms can be helpful as adjuncts to psychotherapy. The therapist, client, and psychiatrist need to evaluate whether any of the drug therapies are desirable and appropriate. A few of these treatments are discussed below.

OPIOID WITHDRAWAL & TREATMENTS

Withdrawal symptoms will begin 6 to 12 hours after the last dose. They usually peak in 48 to 72 hours, then gradually lessen and disappear after 7 to 10 days. Withdrawal from opioids is not life-threatening, whereas withdrawal from barbiturates and alcohol can be.[19] The protracted withdrawal period from opioids often leads patients to self-medicate with other opioid-like drugs to alleviate their discomfort; this leads to a continuation of the addiction.

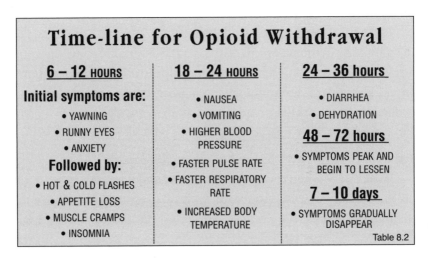

Time-line for Opioid Withdrawal

6 – 12 HOURS	18 – 24 HOURS	24 – 36 hours
Initial symptoms are:	• NAUSEA	• DIARRHEA
• YAWNING	• VOMITING	• DEHYDRATION
• RUNNY EYES	• HIGHER BLOOD PRESSURE	**48 – 72 hours**
• ANXIETY		• SYMPTOMS PEAK AND BEGIN TO LESSEN
Followed by:	• FASTER PULSE RATE	
• HOT & COLD FLASHES	• FASTER RESPIRATORY RATE	**7 – 10 days**
• APPETITE LOSS		• SYMPTOMS GRADUALLY DISAPPEAR
• MUSCLE CRAMPS	• INCREASED BODY TEMPERATURE	
• INSOMNIA		Table 8.2

Clonidine & opioid withdrawal

A general increase in CNS activity is seen during withdrawal from opioids, nicotine, and alcohol. This increase is thought to be due to the action of NE. Clonidine/Catapres (used to treat hypertension) can be helpful in lessening these symptoms. Clonidine inhibits the release of NE, which leads to a decrease in the agitation that usually occurs during withdrawal.

Clonidine is administered either by transdermal skin patch or sublingually (under the tongue). It does not pass through the gastrointestinal tract; this is a major advantage considering the GI disturbances which are frequently present during opioid withdrawal. Clonidine treatment for heroin detoxification takes seven days.[20]

Adverse effects of clonidine

People complain of tiredness and *dysphoria* (feeling bad) during clonidine treatment.[20]

Naltrexone for opioid withdrawal

Naltrexone/Trexan/ReVia is a mixed narcotic antagonist and agonist. Taken orally, it is useful for people who have already been detoxified, and it has been found helpful in preventing relapse. Since it binds strongly to opioid receptors, a person taking naltrexone will not get "high" if opioids are used because the opioid cannot displace the naltrexone at the receptor. Administration of naltrexone will cause withdrawal in someone who is currently addicted to opioids. Agonist (opioid-like) effects are minimal. Taking naltrexone leads to increased production of endorphins, leading to feelings of well-being.[21]

Methadone withdrawal & methadone maintenance

Opioid addicts can receive methadone either as a way to gradually withdraw from opioid use, or as a way to continue using while remaining free from the cycle of crime and the risks associated with illegal drugs, such as infection with HIV or hepatitis C through contaminated needles. These risks are a major public health concern.

Methadone is given in an oral form and dispensed daily through licensed methadone clinics. Methadone is an opioid and causes physical dependency. There will be withdrawal symptoms if a person on methadone decides to decrease the dose or stop taking the drug.[19]

Buprenorphine & opioid withdrawal

Two new formulations are now available for the treatment of withdrawal symptoms seen with opioid dependence. The drug buprenorphine/Subutex is intended for the initial stages of withdrawal, and buprenorphine+naloxone/Suboxone is used during the maintenance phase of treatment. Buprenorphine blocks most of the effects of heroin, which discourages relapse and safeguards against overdose. Buprenorphine causes less sedation and dysphoria than methadone. A patient who is taking buprenorphine+naloxone will be unable to get high if opioids are taken. The main advantage of these compounds is that they are available for patients to take home, eliminating the need to visit a clinic every day, as is required with methadone treatment. Some of the adverse effects are:

- sweating
- nausea
- sleep difficulties
- mood swings
- headaches
- flu-like symptoms[22]

Rapid detox

Rapid detox is a new and controversial drug-detoxification method. It is primarily being used for people addicted to opioids. The treatment can take place over a long weekend and costs about $10,000. The rapid-detox centers claim to have success rates as high as 60% (these claims have not been independently validated) compared to the 15% to 30% success rates for opioid addicts who complete traditional treatment.

A full medical work-up is required before the procedure. The treatment usually takes place in a hospital Intensive Care Unit (ICU) and is overseen by an anesthesiologist with a team of nurses and technicians. This process involves the administration of naltrexone after the patient is under general anesthesia. Because the patient is asleep, there is no conscious experience of the unpleasant symptoms that occur during the initial phase of opioid withdrawal. When the anesthesia wears off the patient is given medication to sleep and goes home the next morning. After treatment, the patient takes naltrexone once a day for up to nine months, or has a naltrexone pellet implanted that lasts for six weeks. If the person does use opioids after the detox treatment, the naltrexone will prevent the experience of getting high. Post-treatment counseling is also usually provided.[23]

Other Treatments for Severe Pain

OXYCODONE + ULTRA-LOW NALTREXONE/OXYTREX

This new drug contains a combination of opioid and ultra-low opioid antagonist compounds and is currently being tested in animals. It is intended to be used as a medication for chronic pain, and is comparable to oxycodone. It is believed that including ultra-low opioid antagonists as part of the formulation will prevent the symptoms of withdrawal that are usually experienced when an opioid is stopped after prolonged use.[24]

ANALGESIC IMPLANTS

Implants allow people with severe pain to receive medication at a constant rate and without interruption. In general, pain medications are more effective, and lower doses are sufficient, if taken before the pain becomes severe. Using implants is also very convenient and avoids the risk of overdose. Narcotic implants are being tested which are placed under the skin and continue to release an analgesic compound for a period of three months. All the other adverse effects of opioids still occur with implants.[15]

NICOTINE ANALOGS

It has been known since the 1930's that nicotine is helpful for relieving pain. Because of its addictive and toxic effects, it is not used routinely in combination with other analgesics. Researchers are exploring the use of analogs to nicotine that are analgesic but do not have the other adverse effects caused by opioids.[25]

DORSAL ROOT SURGERY

Specific nerves carry pain messages from the pelvic organs through a section of spinal cord known as the dorsal column. Cutting this tiny nerve bundle stops most pelvic pain messages from reaching the brain. It is not known yet whether cutting these pathways will deprive the patient of other important functions, or eliminate pain messages that would alert the CNS of a medical problem. Effects of the surgery are often temporary, and pain may return and be even more severe than before. Even with these potential limitations, the surgery is useful for terminally-ill patients in severe pain.[26]

NERVE CELL-DESTROYING TOXINS

Methods are being developed to destroy the nerve cells that transmit chronic-pain messages to the brain. This is done by attaching a toxin to Substance P, a neurotransmitter known to be involved in pain transmission. Substance P carries the toxin to the cells which are transmitting the pain signal, destroying them. Compounds are being tested on animals to see if this method works, and a drug is being sought that does not kill the nerve cells, so that the process could be reversible. The main risk of this method is that sensations other than those of chronic pain could be lost when nerve cells are destroyed.[27]

Direct Relevance to Psychotherapy

The presence of chronic and severe pain, although in itself not life-threatening, leads many people to feelings of helplessness, physical dependence, and frequently to suicidal thoughts and actions. The search continues for compounds to treat severe and chronic pain that do not cause physical dependence; as of this writing, this type of compound has not been found.

Health care providers are beginning to recognize that one way of helping patients with chronic pain is through understanding their personality characteristics. Using the strengths of an individual's personality as an asset will facilitate the treatment of their pain.[4]

Pain medications can decrease a client's access to unconscious or disturbing material, thereby decreasing the effectiveness of psychotherapy. The degree to which therapy is influenced depends upon dose and level of tolerance to the specific drug. Since pain medications are often addictive, it is important to be aware that clients may be currently addicted, in withdrawal, or in recovery from an addiction. All of these conditions will affect psychotherapy, as will severe pain. Psychotherapists are frequently called upon for support and wisdom by clients who are in physical as well as emotional pain, others who are addicted to pain killers, and some who are looking for alternative methods for dealing with their pain. The best way to be of assistance is to be aware of the options available, to discuss these with each client, and to help the client determine which treatment or treatments is likely to be most effective.

References for Chapter 8

1. Ventafridda, V., Bianchi, M., Ripamonti, C., Sacerdote, P., De Conno, F., Zecca, E. & Panerai, A. E., (1990). Studies on the effects of antidepressant drugs on the antinociceptive action of morphine and on plasma morphine in rat and man. *Pain*, 43(2), 155–162.

2. Onghena, P. & Van Houdenhove, B. (1992). Antidepressant-induced analgesia in chronic non-malignant pain: A meta-analysis of 39 placebo-controlled studies. *Pain*, 49(2), 205–219.

3. Ansari, A. (2000). The efficacy of newer antidepressants in the treatment of chronic pain: A review of the current literature. *Harv. Rev. Psychiatry*, 7, 257–277.

4. Gatchel, R. G. & Weisberg, J. N. (2000). *Personality Characteristics of Patients with Pain*. Washington D.C.: American Psychological Association.

5. Joranson, D. E., MSSW, Cleeland, C. S., PhD, Weissman, D. E., MD, & Gilson, A. M., MS. (1992). Opioids for chronic cancer and non-cancer pain: A survey of state medical board members. Retrieved Oct. 12, 2003, from http://www.ampainsoc.org/

6. Day, R. O., Furst, D. E., Graham, G. G. & Champion, G. D. (1987). The clinical pharmacology of aspirin and the salicylates. In: Paulus, H. E., Furst, D. E. & Dromgoole, S. H. Eds. *Anti-inflammatory agents, nonsteroidal, Vol. 16 Drugs for rheumatic disease*. New York: Churchill Livingstone. 227–264.

7. Schlegel, S. I. (1987). General characteristics of nonsteroidal anti-inflammatory drugs. In: Paulus, H. E., Furst, D. E. & Dromgoole, S. H. Eds. *Anti-inflammatory agents, nonsteroidal. Vol. 16. Drugs for rheumatic disease*. New York: Churchill Livingstone. 203–226.

8. Leo, R. J. (2002). *A Concise Guide to Pain Management for Psychiatrists*. Washington, DC.: American Psychiatric Press.

9. Avellanosa, A. N. & West, C. R. (1982). Experience with transcutaneous electrical nerve stimulation for relief of intractable pain in cancer patients. *J. Med.*, 13(3), 203–213.

10. Swerdlow, M. (1984). Anticonvulsant drugs and chronic pain. *Clin. Neuropharm.*, 7(1), 51–82.

11. Fine, P. G. (1993). Nerve blocks, herpes zoster, and postherpetic neuralgia. In: Watson, C. P. N., Ed. *Pain research and clinical management, Vol. 8. Herpes zoster and postherpetic neuralgia*. New York: Elseverir Science Publishers. 173–183.

12. Joshi, J. H., DeJongh, C. A., Schnaper, N., Fortner, C. L. & Wiernik, P. H. (1982). Amphetamine therapy for enhancing the comfort of terminally ill patients with cancer. *18th Annual Meeting of the American Society of Clinical Oncology*, Apr., 25–27.

13. Forrest, W. H., Jr., Brown, B. W., Jr., Brown, C. R., Defaulque, R., Gold, M., Gordon, H. E., James, K. E., Katz, J., Mahler, D. L., Schroff, P. & Teutsch, G. (1977). Dextroamphetamine with morphine for the treatment of postoperative pain. *N. Engl. J. Med.*, 296(13), 712–715.

14. Spiegel, K., Kalb, R. & Pasternak, G. W. (1983). Analgesic activity of tricyclic

antidepressants. *Ann. Neurol.*, 13(4), 462–465.

15. Lazorthes, Y., Verdie, J. C., Bastide, R., Lavados, A. & Descouens, D. (1985). Spinal versus intraventricular chronic opiate administration with implantable drug delivery devices for cancer pain. *Appl. Neurophysiol.*, 48(1–6), 234–241.

16. Mantyh, P. (2000). Understanding substance P and the substance P receptor. Presented at the XXIInd Congress of the Collegium Internationale Neuro-Psychopharmacologicum (CINP); July 10, 2000; Brussels, Belgium. Abstract.

17. Gol, A. (1967). Relief of pain by electrical stimulation of the septal area. *J. Neurol. Sci.*, 5(1), 115–120.

18. Max, M. B., Payne, R., MD, Edwards, W. T., Inturrisi, C. E. & Sunshine, A., MD. (1999). Retrieved Oct. 12, 2003 from http://www.medsch.wisc.edu/painpolicy/publicat/92jmldo.htm, *Principals of analgesic use in the treatment of acute pain and chronic cancer pain. A concise guide to medical practice* (4th ed.). Glenview, IL : American Pain Society.

19. Chiang, W. K., MD & Goldfrank, L. R., MD. (1990). Substance withdrawal. *Emergency Medicine Clinics of North America*, Aug., 8(3), 613–631.

20. Fingerhood, M. I., Thompson, M. R. & Jasinski, D. R. (2001). A comparison of clonidine and buprenorphine in the outpatient treatment of opiate withdrawal. *Substance Abuse*, 22(3), 193–199.

21. Rabinowitz, J., Cohen, H. & Atias, S. (2002). Outcomes of naltrexone maintenance following ultrarapid opiate detoxification versus intensive inpatient detoxification. *Am. J. Addict.*, 11(1), 52–56.

22. Benson, E. (2003). A new treatment for addiction. *Monitor on Psychology*, June, 18–20.

23. Simon, D. L. (2002). Rapid opioid detoxification using opioid antagonists: History, theory and the state of the art. *Perspect. Psychiatr. Care,* 36(4), 113–120.

24. Retrieved Nov. 24, 2003 from http://www.paintherapeutics.com/OxytrexCallfinal.pdf

25. Crooks, P., PhD. (1999). UK Researcher develops nicotinic drugs with R. J. Reynolds. *UK Chandler Medical Center News.* Retrieved Oct. 17, 2003 from http://www.mc.uky.edu/mcpr/news/1999/July/nicotine.htm

26. Simpson, S. (1999). Pain, pain, go away: Snipping a nerve pathway in the spinal cord may bring instant relief. *Science News*, 155, 108–110.

27. Wiley, R. G. & Kline, I. V. R. H. (2000). Neuronal lesioning with axonally transported toxins. *J. Neurosci. Methods,* 103(1), 73–82.

Chapter 9

Consciousness-Altering Drugs

Our normal waking consciousness, rational consciousness as we call it, is but one special type of consciousness, wilst all about it, parted from it by the filmiest of screens, there lie potential forms of consciousness entirely different....No account of the universe in its totality can be final which leaves these other forms of consciousness quite disregarded.

William James

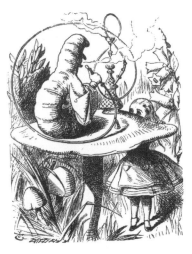

Over the years this group of drugs has been referred to by many different names, including psycholytic, psychotomimetic, empathogenic, and entheogenic, to mention just a few. In 1956, LSD researcher Humphrey Osmond[1] coined the term "psychedelic" (mind-revealing) by combining the Greek roots *psyche* (mind or soul) and *delos* (revealing or manifesting).

There is no one term or phrase that adequately describes the different qualities and effects of the drugs included in this category. The one quality they all share is the ability to dramatically alter consciousness and to change one's experience of reality. These drugs can affect perception, emotions, cognition, and various combinations of these experiences. There is a high degree of unpredictability of response with these drugs. Different people's responses to the same drug may vary, and one person's response to the same drug, taken at different times, may also vary.

Set, setting, drug

This class of drugs is unique in that the nature and intensity of each person's experience is greatly influenced by the set and setting in which the drug is taken. "Set" refers to internal mind set. One's expectations, fears, and previous experiences all influence one's set. "Setting" refers to the external setting in which the drug is taken. The experience will be very different if a drug is taken at a rock concert, in one's home, in a sunny meadow, or in any environment with special significance.[2] As the connections between the mind and body are better understood, it is becoming more widely accepted that responses to many drugs, not only those in this category, are influenced by set and setting. This influence is so great with psychedelics that it is essential to consciously design the set and setting in a way that facilitates one's specific intention or goal for the experience.

Marijuana & Hashish

Marijuana, which refers to the dried leaves and flowering tops of the plants *Cannabis sativa* (C. sativa) and *Cannabis indica* (C. indica), is known by many names. Some examples are pot, weed, reefer, grass, and bhang. Hashish, often called "hash," is made from the resin that forms at the plant's flowering tips.[3]

Cannabis has a long history as a medicinal plant and has been used in many cultures for treating a variety of ailments. In the United States, the widespread use of cannabis compounds for medical purposes is well-documented, and it was a standard entry in the *U.S. Pharmacopia* until it was removed from the 1942 edition after the criminalization of its use in 1937.[4] There has been renewed interest in its medicinal uses since about 1971, and the controversy over its value as a medicine, and its danger as a drug of abuse, continues to rage in America. Many states have decriminalized it for medical use, but under the Controlled Substances Act of 1970 the Department of Justice has defined it as Schedule I drug,[5] a narcotic with a high potential for abuse and no accepted medical value (the same classification as heroin). Despite government assertions, many doctors believe it has valid medical uses and is especially effective for:

- improving appetite
- reducing intraoccular pressure of glaucoma
- relieving nausea resulting from chemotherapy
- decreasing nausea from medications used to treat HIV [6]

There is evidence that marijuana can be used as part of treatment for alcohol, heroin, and amphetamine dependence.[7,8] More than nine million people over the age of 12 in the U.S. use marijuana every year, and one percent of Americans smoke marijuana daily.[9]

Marijuana is unique in that it has stimulant, sedative, and hallucinogenic effects. The specific type of effect one gets is strongly influenced by the dose. Cannabis contains over 400 compounds, many of which are psychoactive. The main psychoactive compound is delta-9-tetrahydrocannabinol (THC).[6]

Route of administration

The most common route of administration in the U.S. is via the lungs by smoking. When marijuana is smoked, the blood in the lungs absorbs the THC and transports it to the brain. The peak of intensity occurs soon after ingestion. Marijuana can also be absorbed through the GI tract when eaten (usually in cookies or brownies). Absorption is much slower than when smoked, and the effects may continue to increase for two to three hours after eating. Due to the slow rate of absorption, it is much more difficult to control the dose with this method of ingestion. If marijuana is smoked, most symptoms are usually gone after a few hours; if eaten, symptoms last longer.[10]

Metabolism

Marijuana is metabolized primarily by the liver. Because THC is fat-soluble, it is excreted very slowly. One week after ingestion, 25% to 30% of the THC consumed remains in the body. Traces of marijuana may be detectable for as long as 30 days after ingestion.[10]

PHYSICAL & COGNITIVE EFFECTS OF MARIJUANA INTOXICATION

The common symptoms of marijuana intoxication are:

- a state of euphoria
- feelings of relaxation
- sense of time slowing down
- enhanced sensitivity to humor
- alienation
- feelings of paranoia
- difficulty concentrating
- feeling remote and withdrawn
- short-term impairment of memory [6, 9, 10]

Physiological changes–acute

The acute effect of THC on the respiratory system is one of bronchodialation (opening of bronchial tubes). There is a dose-dependent decrease in cognitive and psychomotor performance. At higher doses, driving can be impaired. [6, 9, 10] THC also causes:

- red eyes
- increased appetite
- decreased salivation
- lower skin temperature
- an increase in heart rate
- decreased intraoccular pressure

Physiological changes–long-term

Alteration of sleep architecture is seen with marijuana use. REM sleep decreases, Stage 4 sleep increases, and total sleep time increases. [6, 9, 10]

Tolerance

Tolerance to the effects of cannabis develops with daily use. A mild physical dependence also develops. People often smoke cannabis to decrease anxiety; over time, higher doses are needed to obtain this effect. [10]

Withdrawal

Symptoms of cannabis withdrawal are the opposite of those that occur with intoxication. Some of these are:

- restlessness
- anorexia
- vomiting
- tremors
- irritability
- diarrhea
- nausea
- disturbed sleep

These symptoms are seen when any drug with a sedating effect is withdrawn after someone has become habituated to it. Interestingly, some people who have smoked marijuana daily for years do not become physically dependent. Men are more likely than women to become dependent, and adolescents are at greater risk than adults.[10]

Antimotivational syndrome

This syndrome defines a pattern of personality changes that has been noted in some daily users. Symptoms are:

- general loss of motivation
- apathy • lack of concern for the future

Some of the symptoms persist long after the drug's effects have worn off and may include:

- loss of ambition
- impaired memory
- loss of effectiveness
- difficulty in concentrating
- diminished ability to carry out long-term plans

All these symptoms lead to a decline in work or school performance. It usually takes several weeks after the marijuana use is stopped before the syndrome disappears completely.[10]

There is controversy over whether marijuana is the cause of this syndrome, or whether marijuana is used to alleviate symptoms of depression. The question is: does the antimotivational syndrome reflect symptoms of an underlying depression, or are the symptoms being caused by the use of marijuana?[10]

Effects of marijuana on the respiratory system

With long-term use, inflammatory changes take place in the lung tissue causing obstructive pulmonary disease. This process eventually leads to a decrease in one's ability to get air into the lungs (bronchoconstriction). Anyone with a breathing disorder (e.g., asthma, bronchitis, emphysema) who smokes marijuana will experience a worsening of the disorder over time.[9, 10]

The U.S. government prohibits the possession of marijuana, and there are no regulations governing its safe cultivation; therefore, marijuana obtained "on the street" may contain unknown contaminants and pesticides. In contrast to a cigarette, a marijuana "joint" is usually smoked down very far or consumed completely, leading to ingestion of more of the tars, which contributes significantly to lung cancer. The typical joint has more hydrocarbons that cause cancer than are found in cigarettes.

Effects of marijuana on sexual functioning

Marijuana can affect sexual functioning in various ways. Some claim that marijuana has aphrodisiac qualities and causes an enhancement of the sexual experience. This may be due to a decrease in anxiety, an increased enhancement of the senses, or both. Studies show that smoking marijuana causes a suppression of testicular function, and may also suppress ovarian function. These effects are relevant for anyone who wants to conceive a child and for anyone with known fertility problems.[9]

Other effects of marijuana

Women of childbearing age need to be made aware that during pregnancy the THC molecule crosses the placental barrier and passes into the bloodstream of the fetus. THC is also found in the breast milk of nursing mothers.

Studies have shown that marijuana may be harmful to patients who are immunocompromised. This is of particular concern for HIV patients or anyone who has an autoimmune disease.[9] The potentially harmful compounds include:

- cannabinoids
- pyrolyzed gasses
- particulate matter
- contaminants (adulterants, pesticides, various fungi and their metabolites)[9]

Psychological treatment for marijuana users

Many modalities of therapy have been tried with habitual users who want to stop. These include: family therapy, community reinforcement programs, cognitive, behavioral and motivational treatments, and therapy supplemented with discussions of family dynamics. All the treatment strategies are equally successful. One year after completion, all modalities of treatment show success rates about 30% better than control groups receiving no treatment.[10]

Lysergic Acid Diethylamide (LSD, "acid")

Historically, LSD-like compounds may have been derived from grain infected with a fungus called "wheat rust" that develops on wheat and rye. This naturally-occurring fungus contains ergot compounds which dilate blood vessels, and in high doses, can result in bleeding disorders. Ingesting infected grain causes a potentially fatal disease known as *St. Anthony's Fire*. The symptoms are burning sensations in the hands and feet, and hallucinations. High doses of ergot can lead to extensive internal bleeding.[11]

There are hints that a compound like LSD was part of the annual rituals known as the Eleusinian Mysteries which were practiced in ancient Greece for 2,000 years. The participants were not allowed to talk about what went on in the rituals, hence "mysteries." Pottery has survived from this period which is decorated with paintings of the goddess of the harvest, Demeter, holding sheaves of wheat. This may support the idea that wheat infected with an ergot compound was used in the rites. What took place at Eleusis is unknown, and experts differ as to what specific compound, if any, was involved in the rites.[12]

History of LSD

In 1943, Dr. Albert Hofmann was working as a research chemist at Sandoz Pharmaceutical Laboratories in Switzerland. He was searching for a compound to act as a "blood stimulant," using ergot derivatives because of their known action on blood vessels. He would sometimes try compounds on himself, as scientists often do. Most drugs are active at doses ranging from one milligram to hundreds of milligrams, so when he took a mere 250 *micrograms* of LSD (.25 mg), he believed it was a minute dose (for almost any other drug, it would be). Hofmann soon discovered that 250 micrograms of LSD caused a potent and long-lasting change in his perceptual and emotional state.[13]

LSD is effective in doses as low as 50 micrograms (.05 mg), and its effects (popularly called a "trip") last 12 to 16 hours after a single dose. It may be that a metabolite of LSD, and not the LSD itself, causes the changes in perception and feelings. Or, taking LSD may lead to a series of changes in the CNS which then lead to its effects.[14] Estimates are that 13.2 million Americans over age 12 have tried LSD at least once (up from 8.1 million in 1985).[15, 16]

Effects of LSD

The LSD experience varies greatly from person to person. Factors of set, setting, and the amount of the drug taken, all influence the experience. Frequently, there is an alteration of perception and feeling which can range in intensity from very mild to extreme. Depending on many factors, the experience may also vary from wildly ecstatic to utterly hellish. Many of the factors that can influence expectations, such as personal history, state of mind, and reports by friends, are difficult to quantify.[2, 15]

Tolerance to LSD

With daily use, tolerance to LSD will develop in two to four days.

Although some psychological dependence may develop, there are no signs of physical dependence with long-term or repeated use. Cross-tolerance develops between LSD, mescaline, and psilocybin.[13] These compounds have different chemical structures, but all have similar psychedelic effects. The cross-tolerance hints that there may be a common metabolic pathway or a common end-point for these drugs.

Toxic reaction to LSD

There are no adverse physical effects due to ingesting even very large amounts of LSD, although there have been many reports of extremely upsetting psychological experiences. Intensity of experience is related to size of dose, but there is no direct relationship between the dose and whether the experience will be pleasant or terrifying. Taking LSD may uncover unconscious fears or fantasies that may be undesirable and frightening. The unpleasant symptoms most frequently reported are paranoia, delusions, and agitation.[15]

People with an affective disorder or schizophrenia may become mentally disorganized after taking LSD, and their symptoms may not clear when the LSD has worn off. In cases where symptoms continue long afterward, diagnosis and treatment for the underlying disorder is appropriate.[15]

Antianxiety drugs (BZs in particular) can be given for agitation. Some people report that taking large doses of vitamins B and C also can be helpful in counteracting the effects of LSD. All of the effects usually are gone within 24 hours, and the normal state of consciousness is regained.[14]

LSD psychotherapy

The use of LSD as an aid to psychotherapy has been studied extensively by Stan Grof and his colleagues and is explored in detail in his book, *LSD Psychotherapy* (1980). The researchers found that using LSD as an adjunct to psychotherapy lessened defenses and allowed access to affective experiences and memories that had previously not been available to the conscious mind.[17]

Prior to its criminalization, LSD was used experimentally to create what was called a "functional psychosis." This state mimicked a psychotic state, but was drug-induced and time-limited. It was hoped that the ability to create a psychotic state under experimental conditions would increase understanding and yield information that could be used in developing new treatment methods. This research was discontinued in the U.S. after 1966 due to legal restrictions.[17]

Dimethyltryptamine (DMT)

DMT occurs naturally in some South American plants and is used in shamanic practices throughout the Amazon basin. The usual forms of administration are via the nasal membranes by snorting, through the lungs by smoking, and by sprinkling the compounds onto marijuana and then smoking. All of these methods cause an immediate onset of effects. The DMT experience usually lasts for about 30 minutes, after which the user returns to a normal state. DMT is sometimes said to have effects like short-acting LSD. It causes vivid visual hallucinations and sometimes a loss of awareness of one's surroundings.[18] It can be described as "going to the peak of an intense LSD experience in the time it takes to exhale." For anyone who is not both familiar with the LSD experience, and comfortable with it, this can be extremely disorienting and frightening.

Phenylethylamines

It is said that MDA and similar drugs can be synthesized from two oils derived from nutmeg, safrol and myristicin. Nutmeg is referred to as a narcotic fruit in the *Atharva Veda* (one of a small number of ancient Indian texts that deals with healing and prolonging life).

Some examples of phenylethylamines are:

- methylenedioxyamphetamine (MDA)
- methylenedioxymethamphetamine (MDMA, "ecstasy," "X")
- 3-methoxy-4,5-methylenedioxyphenylisopropylamine (MMDA)
- 3,4,5-trimethoxyphenethylamine (mescaline/peyote)

They all are structurally similar to DA, NE, and the amphetamines.

Before 1985, it was legal to use phenylethylamines to facilitate psychotherapy. In *The Healing Journey,* Claudio Naranjo wrote about the use of MDA and MMDA in conjunction with psychotherapy. He calls these drugs "feeling enhancers." They are also called "empathogens," a designation for drugs that enhance empathy. When his patients were under the influence of one of these compounds, Naranjo observed an intensification of feeling, access to underlying experiences, and spontaneous age-regression.[19]

METHYLENEDIOXYAMPHETAMINE (MDMA)

MDMA ("ecstasy") has become popular as a "club drug" at dance events known as "raves." MDMA is believed to induce feelings of love, decrease fear,[20] and facilitate the "working through" of psychological material by reducing defenses. Before it became illegal, many psychotherapists were using MDMA to facilitate psychotherapy.[21]

MDMA causes the release of all stored 5-HT from the vesicles of the nerve cell. The reuptake of the released 5-HT is blocked.[22]

Mushrooms, Peyote, & Ayahuasca

PSILOCYBIN MUSHROOMS

Stropharia cubensis is the mushroom most frequently used during shamanic rituals by Native Americans in the U.S. and Mexico to attain an altered state of awareness. The mushrooms, which usually grow on the dung of deer or cattle, are used in religious ceremonies for divination, and by shamans in healing ceremonies. Considered sacred for 3,000 years, they are depicted in stone sculptures found in

Guatemala dating from around 1000 BCE.

The main active ingredient is psilocybin (4-phosphoryloxy-N,N-dimethyltryptamine); an accompanying compound, psilocin (4-hydroxyl-N,N-dimethyltryptamine) is also present in much smaller amounts. Psilocybin, which is in the chemical group called indolealkylamines, is similar in molecular structure to 5-HT. [23]

Effects of psilocybin

Ingesting these mushrooms causes fundamental alterations in consciousness, including changes in the perception of time, space, and in both the psychic and bodily selves. The sense of being an objective observer to oneself ("being on the outside looking in") is sometimes experienced. This experience of objectivity can lead to insights into one's motives and behaviors that are not accessible during ordinary consciousness. Sight and hearing are greatly enhanced; this may be experienced as exaggerations in perception, or as auditory and visual hallucinations. Also enhanced is the ability to clearly recall long-forgotten events, often from early childhood.[23]

FLY AGARIC MUSHROOM

Amanita muscarina is native to Lapland, Siberia, and other regions in extreme northern latitudes and is used by Sami and Siberian shamans in their healing practices. The active ingredients in this mushroom are muscimole and muscarine. Researcher Gordon Wasson has investigated them extensively and believes they are the Soma known by ancient Indo-Europeans as the "mushroom of immortality." [23]

These mushrooms have consciousness-changing ability whether eaten raw, cooked, or dried. Because of the way the ingredients are metabolized, the urine of someone or some animal that has ingested the mushroom is stronger in narcotic and intoxicating properties than the unmetabolized mushrooms. Shamans often drink the urine of an intoxicated person, their own urine, or the urine of a reindeer that had eaten the mushrooms.[23]

Effects of amanita

The effects begin 15 to 20 minutes after ingestion and last for a few hours. First the person sleeps for about two hours. This is not a normal sleep, as one cannot be roused from it. There is an awareness of external sounds and an experience of colored visions. After awakening, people report a feeling of elation that lasts from three to four hours. During this period, people report a capacity for feats of extraordinary physical strength, and find this very enjoyable. Shamans believe that the mushrooms will tell anyone who eats them what ails them when they are sick, explain a dream, show them the upper or underground world, or foretell the future.[23]

PEYOTE

The peyote cactus (*Lophophora williamsii*) is native to an area ranging from about the Rio Grande river and extending south between Mexico's eastern and western Sierra Madre mountain ranges to the Tropic of Cancer. Pre-Columbian art, dating from approximately 100 BCE, depicts the peyote cactus. Today, peyote is used in the shamanic practices of the Huichol Indians and is a sacrament of the Native American Church.[7]

Effects of mescaline

The main psychoactive compound in peyote is mescaline (3,4,5-trimethoxyphenethylamine). Peyote is very bitter and difficult to swallow by itself and is usually ingested as a tea, swallowed in capsules, or ground-up and mixed with food. About 45 minutes after ingestion, most people begin to see brilliantly colored images, particularly geometric designs, and "auras," which appear as halos of light around people and objects. There is an enhancement of auditory, olfactory, gustatory, and tactile sensations. There are feelings of weightlessness, as well as the experience of macroscopia (the ability to observe things with the details greatly magnified, such as watching a candle burning, or ice melting). There is an alteration of one's perception of time and space; time seems to move more slowly, and objects appear to change size.[24]

Most people report less cognitive distortion with peyote than with LSD, and because of this there are fewer anxious reactions. This may be related to size of the dose rather than to the specific compound. Peyote is often taken in a religious or spiritual setting. The use of ritual, and having elders present to guide the session, are factors that decrease fear.[24]

AYAHUASCA

Ayahuasca is always a combination of at least two main plant substances: The *Banisteriopsis caapi* vine, which contains harmaline (an MAO inhibitor), and the *Psychotria viridis*, a green, leafy plant which contains the vision-inducing DMT or other tryptamine. The hallucinogenic extract has a variety of names, including ayahuasca, caapi, natema, pinde, and yajé.[18]

Effects of harmaline

- nausea
- dizziness
- general malaise
- numbness of the hands, feet, and face
- visions (considered useful in divination)

Unlike some experiences with other psychedelic drugs, neither color enhancement nor distortions of body image are present.[18]

Harmaline overdose

In large doses harmaline causes tremors and clonic (jerking) convulsions. With toxic doses harmaline causes:

- respiratory arrest
- fall in body temperature
- a weakening of cardiac muscles which results in a vasodepressant effect

The effects are related to the capacity of these compounds to inhibit monoamine oxidase.

Dissociative Anesthetics

Phencyclidine, Ketamine, and dextromethorphan are in a group of drugs classified as dissociative anesthetics due to the frequent "out of body" experiences reported by users, and the numbing of physical sensation that accompanies intoxication. These drugs have some depressant effect on respiration and blood pressure, but much less than other anesthetics.[25] Because dextromethorphan has been added to the drugs in this class, they are now being called "dissociatives."

PHENCYCLIDINE (PCP)

Until recently the main drug of abuse in this category was PCP ("angel dust"). It was originally developed in the 1950's as an intravenous surgical anesthetic. It was never approved for human use because of feelings of delirium and agitation that were experienced by test subjects emerging from the PCP anesthesia. PCP can be taken orally, or mixed with marijuana or tobacco and smoked.[15]

Effects of PCP

Depending on the dose taken and the route of administration, PCP can have hallucinogenic, analgesic, stimulant, and/or depressive effects. A behavioral tolerance develops with chronic use. Although there is no development of physical dependence, a psychological dependence can develop. There will be no physical withdrawal symptoms if use is discontinued. Symptoms such as memory-loss and depression may persist for as long as a year after a chronic user stops taking PCP.[25]

Although the half-life of PCP is only 45 minutes, traces of the drug may stay in the body up to three days due to its fat-solubility. In low doses, PCP acts as a CNS depressant. Taking less than a 5 milligram dose causes a state similar to alcohol intoxication. With doses in the 5 mg to 10 mg range, PCP may cause *hyperreflexia* (increased muscle tone), and *catalepsy* (cessation of motion and nonresponsiveness to external stimuli, as in catatonic states).[25]

PCP intoxication can induce psychotic symptoms that may persist long after the drug has been metabolized, sometimes for months. Psychotic symptoms occur more frequently in people who have a history of mental illness. In these cases, it is important to determine and to treat the underlying mental disorder (usually with antipsychotic medication).[25]

Treatment for PCP intoxication

People who have taken PCP often appear agitated and violent. For this reason, it is very important to calm the person as much as possible. This is best accomplished by decreasing external stimuli (putting the person in a dark, quiet room). Emergency room personnel sometimes use restraints to prevent these patients from harming themselves or others. A BZ such as diazepam is often used to decrease the agitation and muscle hypertonicity. Most symptoms of the intoxication will clear in several hours.[25]

PCP overdose

Symptoms of overdose can occur with a dose of 20 mg or more. Overdose may cause a hypertensive crisis, seizures, and a respiratory depression that can lead to a comatose state. This coma can last for several days and can be fatal. The patient must be hospitalized to establish adequate oxygen intake and for treatment of the hypertension. Diazepam or one of the other BZs is usually given to decrease the possibility of seizures.[25]

KETAMINE

Ketamine ("vitamin K") was developed in 1963 as a general anesthetic for use during surgery. It is most useful for patients who have respiratory conditions that would put them at increased risk if barbiturates, or most other types of general anesthesia, were used. Ketamine is useful with the pediatric and elderly populations due to the large individual metabolic variations in these groups, which makes the correct dose of anesthetic more difficult to calculate.[15]

Although Ketamine is legal to use as an anesthetic, it is not widely used by medical personnel due to fear of having to deal with what is termed "emergence phenomena," the altered states of consciousness experienced as the Ketamine wears off.[15] If not prepared beforehand for what they might experience, patients may become frightened and hard to manage. For this reason, Ketamine is rarely used as a general anesthetic with humans. Since it is very safe, it is often used by veterinarians for surgery on animals.

When used as a recreational drug, Ketamine can be taken by intramuscular injection, snorted, or smoked. Its usual effects are feelings of disembodiment, feeling part of the cosmic energy field, and having colorful visions. There is not much effect on the emotions, and it generally does not provoke fear. The experience usually lasts about an hour.[15]

Other uses for Ketamine

Ketamine is useful for some severe pain syndromes such as the pain of post-herpetic neuralgia. There is evidence that it may be useful with patients who have terminal illnesses to help them overcome their fear of death.[26] Scientists in Russia have been researching the use of Ketamine in conjunction with psychotherapy as a treatment for alcohol and heroin addiction. They have found that psychedelic doses of Ketamine led to a significant rate of abstinence and reduced the craving for heroin.[8]

DEXTROMETHORPHAN (DXM)

DXM ("robo") is a cough-suppressing ingredient found in many over-the-counter cold and cough preparations such as Coricidin and Robitussin. In very high doses, DXM can induce experiences of dissociation that may last for up to six hours. Its mechanism of action is similar to PCP and Ketamine.[15]

Direct Relevance to Psychotherapy

People of all generations regularly use alcohol, and many who grew up in the 1960's and 1970's experimented extensively with psychedelics and marijuana, and more than a few continue to use these drugs and others, either regularly or intermittently. In addition, a significant percentage of the generation now in their twenties and thirties has taken MDMA, Ketamine, and other psychedelics.

Many clients will talk about their drug experiences if they do not receive a negative or judgmental reaction from the therapist. Since these drugs are used so widely, particularly by some populations, it is important that psychotherapists have both an openness to, and an understanding of, the use and effects of the various consciousness-altering drugs. As people mature into their teens, twenties, and thirties, it is common that many will experiment with various drugs as a part of their explorations as to who they are and who they want to be. Psychotherapists need to be proactive in exploring whether their clients are experimenting with drugs.

Most clients will be alert for any hint of judgement or condemnation on the part of the therapist. The ability to stay open and curious to a client's experiences will prove to be the most fruitful approach to gleaning information as to the client's experimentation with, or regular use of, these substances. This openness will allow the therapist and the client to explore, in the therapeutic setting, the meaning and purpose of the client's experiences.

References for Chapter 9

1. Hoffer, A. & Osmond, H. (1967). *The hallucinogens*. New York: Academic Press.
2. Leary. T., Litwin, G. & Metzner, R. (1963). Reactions to psilocybin administered in a supportive environment. *J. Nervous and Mental Disease*, 137, 561–573.
3. Bloomquist, E. R. (1971). *Marijuana: The second trip*. (Rev. ed.) Beverly Hills: Glencoe Press. p. 14–15.
4. Whitebread, C. (1995). The history of the non-medical use of drugs in the United States. A speech to the California Judges Association Annual Conference. Retrieved Dec. 17, 2003 from, http://www.druglibrary.org/schaffer/history/whiteb1.htm
5. Fiano, R. A. (2000). DEA Congressional Testimony, Caucus on International Narcotics Control. July 25, US Dept. of Justice, Drug Enforcement Administration.
6. Zimmer, L. & Morgan, J. P. (1997). *Marijuana myths, marijuana facts: Review of the scientific evidence*. New York, NY: The Lindesmith Center.
7. McClusky, J. (1997). Native American Church peyotism and treatment of alcoholism. *MAPS Bulletin*, VII(4), 3–4.
8. Krupitsky, E., Burakov, A, Romanova, T., Dunaevsky, I. & Strassman, R. (2002). Ketamine psychotherapy for heroin addiction: Immediate effects and follow-up. *J. Subst. Abuse. Treatment*, 23(4), 273–283.
9. Hall, W. (1995). *Project on health implications of cannabis use: A comparative appraisal of health and psychological consequences of alcohol, cannabis, nicotine and opiate use, II. The probable effects of cannabis use*. WHO (World Health Organization). Retrieved Sept. 7, 2003 from www.druglibrary.org/shaffer/hemp/general/who-index.htm.
10. Selden, B. S. MD, Clark, R. F. MD & Curry, S. C. MD. (1990). Marijuana. *Emergency Medicine Clinics of North America*, 8(3), 527–539.
11. *The Merck manual of diagnosis and therapy* (17th ed.). (2001). Rahway, NJ: Merck Sharp & Dohme Research Laboratories.
12. Wasson, R. G., Kramrisch, S., Ott, J. & Ruck, C. (1988). *Persephone's quest: Entheogens and the origins of religion*. New Haven, CT: Yale University Press.
13. Hofmann, A. (1980). *LSD-my problem child, reflections on sacred drugs, mysticism, and science*. New York: McGraw-Hill.
14. Kulig, K., MD. (1990). LSD. *Emergency Medicine Clinics of North America*, 8(3), 551–558.
15. National Institute on Drug Abuse (NIDA). (2001). Hallucinogens and dissociative drugs: Including LSD, PCP, ketamine, dextromethorphan. *NIH Publication,* Number 01–409.
16. US Department of Justice, Drug Enforcement Administration. (1993). LSD in the United States.
17. Grof, S. (1980). *LSD psychotherapy.* Pomona, CA: Hunter House.
18. Metzner, R., PhD. (Ed.) (1999). *Ayahuasca: Human consciousness and the spirits of nature*. New York: Thunder's Mouth Press.
19. Naranjo, Claudio, C. (1974). *The healing journey*. New York: Pantheon Books.

20. Teter, C. J. & Guthrie, S. K. (2001). A comprehensive review of MDMA and GHB: Two common club drugs. *Pharmacotherapy*, 21, 1487–1513.
21. Adamson, S. (1984). *Through the gateway of the heart*. San Francisco, CA: Four Trees Publications.
22. Solowij, N. (1993). Ecstasy (3,4-methylenedioxymethamphetamine). *Current Opinion in Psychiatry*, 6, 411–415.
23. Wasson, R. G. (1980). *The Wondrous Mushroom*. New York: McGraw-Hill.
24. Schultes, R. E. & Hofmann, A. (1979) *Plants of the gods: Origins of hallucinogenic use*. New York: Alfred van der Marck Editions.
25. Baldridge, E. B., MD & Bessen, H. A., MD. (1990). Phencyclidine. *Emergency Medicine Clinics of North America*, 8(3), 541–550.
26. Jansen, K. L. R. (1996). Using ketamine to induce the near-death experience: Mechanism of action and therapeutic potential. *Yearbook for Ethnomedicine and the Study of Consciousness* (Jahrbuch fur Ethnomedizin und Bewubtseinsforschung). Issue 4, 55–81. C. Ratsch; J. R. Baker, (Eds.), Berlin: VWB.

Chapter 10

Cognition-Enhancing Drugs

The term "nootropic" (acting on the mind) is used to describe a relatively new class of drugs which are chemically unrelated and have diverse pharmacological properties. In the past, when the average life span was only until the mid-forties, there was little need for cognition-enhancing drugs. But now as the baby-boom generation ages and the World War II generation lives into their nineties and even longer, interest and demand for this group of drugs is rapidly increasing.

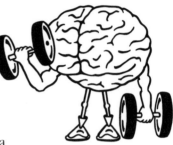

The extension of life that comes with modern medicine brings with it a substantial increase in the geriatric population and the need to treat the diseases of the elderly. Of particular concern are the dementias seen in this population. Growing in tandem with the ever-increasing knowledge about the structural and metabolic changes that take place with aging and contribute to dementia is the rapid development and testing of new drugs and herbal remedies to treat it.[1]

Many of these drugs are designed to improve the memory processes of consolidation, retrieval, and learning. Researchers are trying to develop drugs that improve memory and at the same time avoid the adverse effects, such as insomnia, anorexia, and nervousness, that are caused by many of the drugs that stimulate the CNS.

Some drugs that may delay the onset of *Alzheimer's* disease or that have shown some therapeutic value with patients already affected by Alzheimer's are:

- antioxidants (vitamin C and E, selegiline/Eldepryl)
- hormone replacement therapy (estrogens and/or androgens)

- anti-inflammatory drugs (NSAIDs, e.g. ibuprofen/Motrin, and COX-2 inhibitors, e.g. celecoxib/Celebrex)
- neurotropic agents (human nerve growth factor)
- cholinergic agents (e.g., galantamine/Reminyl)
- cholinesterase inhibitors (rivastigmine/Exelon, donepezil/Aricept, tacrine/Cognex, huperzine)
- statin drugs (lower cholesterol)
- nicotine (stimulates ACh)
- *Ginkgo biloba* (increases blood flow into the CNS)
- phosphotidylserine/PtdSer (a fat-soluble nutrient found naturally in our bodies)
- antiamyloid treatments (gene therapy or vaccines)[1-5]

As this list indicates, many drugs are now being tested for safety and efficacy for the treatment or prevention of Alzheimer's and other forms of dementia. It is hoped that some of these compounds will prove to be effective and have a low toxicity. Since the majority of drugs for dementia have been put on the market very recently, or are still in the testing stage, long-term effects are not yet known.

Alzheimer's Disease

Alzheimer's is a progressive, degenerative disease of the brain which affects approximately four million Americans, three million of whom are living at home and being cared for by family members. If no cure is found, the number of people afflicted with Alzheimer's is expected to double by the year 2050.[6]

The major known risk factors are heredity (although only between 2% and 10% of Alzheimer's patients have the gene for the disease), and head trauma. A moderate concussion in one's medical history doubles the risk of developing Alzheimer's, and a severe concussion more than quadruples the risk. Ten percent of people over age 65 have Alzheimer's, and about 50% of people over the age of 85 are affected.[6]

Symptoms of Alzheimer's disease

The symptoms are similar to other dementias and include:

- impaired ability to reason
- problems with memory (especially recent memory)
- eventual loss of control of the physical body and the ability to speak and care for oneself [6]

Any client who mentions memory problems severe enough to interfere with daily life needs an evaluation for dementia. This can be accomplished with a mini-mental status exam (MMSE) or a test called the 7-Minute Screen (advertised as being able to diagnose the presence of Alzheimer's with a 90% accuracy rate).

Memory difficulties often cause compliance problems with medication. This can lead to other medical problems and drug toxicities that may escalate into greater memory difficulties and even more severe medical problems.

Diagnosis of Alzheimer's disease

The diagnosis of Alzheimer's requires the finding of characteristic "plaques and tangles" using microscopic examination of brain tissue at autopsy. It is believed that the plaques and tangles interfere with the normal functioning of nerve cells and with the production of ACh. Some people who had no signs of dementia have been found to have plaques and tangles. The cause of the plaques and tangles is not fully understood, and there is no known cure for Alzheimer's. Treatments are only minimally effective in stopping the progress of the disease.

It is only through very recent information gained by the use of Positron Emission Tomography (PET) scans and other brain-imaging techniques, specifically functional Magnetic Resonance Imaging (fMRI), that the mystery of Alzheimer's is beginning to be understood. Diagnosis has usually been made by a process of elimination of other types of dementia, and is only 100% definitive at autopsy. Recent studies using PET and fMRI scans indicate that progressive loss of brain cells, particularly in the area of the hippocampus, can be seen by comparing an individual's brain scans over time. There are hopes that these scanning techniques will lead to earlier diagnosis, earlier treatment, and to a better prognosis for those who are at increased risk as well as for those who are already showing early signs of Alzheimer's.[7, 8]

Drug & Herbal Treatments for Dementia

Drugs used to treat dementia are usually in two categories:

1. Drugs aimed at treating the pathological structural changes in the CNS.
2. Drugs aimed at correcting the biochemical changes, specifically the decrease in ACh in the hippocampus.

Ergoloid mesylates

Hydergine is the brand name for a group of compounds (ergot mesylates) which are believed to improve cognition by enhancing the metabolic activity of brain cells. Hydergine is widely used in countries outside the U.S. for the treatment of dementia and cognitive deficits that may accompany aging. It is approved by the FDA for treatment of Alzheimer's disease and has been administered in the U.S. for this purpose since the 1980's. A recent review of the literature concludes that Hydergine shows significant effectiveness when compared with a placebo (although there is some skepticism among authorities in the field about the validity of the research).[9]

Ginkgo biloba

Ginkgo has been widely used outside the U.S. for many years as a brain-energizing herb and to improve memory. Most studies indicate significant cognitive improvement in people who have been taking ginkgo. There are few adverse effects (see pps. 159-160). However, in contrast to the earlier studies, a recent study in people with dementia who took ginkgo either for 12 or 24 weeks showed no significant effect on cognitive decline or any other measurable outcomes compared with a control group taking no medication.[10]

Other herbs

Many herbs are being investigated for nootropic properties. Some that are under study, but are not yet approved by the FDA, are:

- *Bacopa monnieri*/Bacopa
- *Cordyceps sinensis*/Cordyceps
- *Huperzia serrata*/Huperzine A
- *Vinca minor* (periwinkle)/Vinpocetine [11, 12]

Antibiotic therapy

Evidence exists that an accumulation of copper and zinc in the brain promotes the accumulation of beta-amyloid, which may lead to the development of the "plaques" seen in Alzheimer's. The antibiotic clioquinol, which has the ability to chelate metals (form specific molecular complexes), may be able to facilitate removal of copper and zinc from the brain. This may lead to a reduction of amyloid deposits. It is hypothesized that a reduction in amyloid will lead to a decrease of some symptoms of dementia.[13]

Gene therapy

There has been some success in assessing the possibility of repairing brain cells that are no longer producing ACh. This research uses a virus as a vector to insert a gene into brain cells which will then be able to deliver human nerve growth factor. The growth factor nourishes brain cells, and might possibly reverse the neurological changes caused by Alzheimer's. This research is still in the early stages.[14]

Enzyme-blocking therapy

Scientists have identified an enzyme, beta secretase, which is believed to play a role in the buildup of abnormal amyloid plaques. Other researchers are studying the blocking of gamma secretase, another component in the formation of plaques. At this stage it is not known whether there will be any serious detrimental effects caused by blocking either beta or gamma secretase.[15]

Plaque-blocking vaccine

Recently a "vaccine" consisting of beta-amyloid protein has been shown to prevent naturally-occurring amyloid from forming in the brains of lab rats, and to eliminate pre-existing amyloid plaques.[16]

Ampakines

The ampakines are a newly-developed class of drugs which interact with glutamate receptors. Since glutamate is usually excitatory, the theory is that the ampakines may protect cells in the CNS from damage caused by over-stimulation. Ampakines have been found to improve memory and cognition in the elderly.

A profile of the behavioral changes produced by ampakine interaction with AMPA-type glutamate receptors has been established. These changes lead to improvement in certain types of memory, and an increased ability to do tasks of daily living. Ampakine therapy has been shown to enhance memory encoding in humans. Giving ampakines to patients who were suffering from both schizophrenia and Alzheimer's disease has uncovered a synergistic interaction between ampakines and antipsychotic drugs. The first ampakine, Ampalex, is in clinical trials and could be on the market by 2008.[17]

N-methyl-D-aspartate (NMDA) inhibitors

Another theory that attributes Alzheimer's disease to an over-stimulation of certain CNS nerve cells, and that the over-stimulation leads to cell death, has resulted in the development of a compound that works as an antagonist at the NMDA receptors. When these receptors malfunction, there is over-stimulation of nerve cells leading to cell damage and cell death. One compound in this category, memantine hydrochloride/Namenda, is currently available. It is believed to work by providing protection from over-stimulation. Studies indicate an improvement in memory of Alzheimer's patients after 12 weeks. It seems to protect the brain from damage while still allowing normal signal transmission between cells.[18]

Modulatory receptors

A new family of modulatory receptors called metabotropic glutamate (mGlu) receptors has been discovered. The mGlu receptors fine-tune neuronal signaling in CNS circuits. It is thought that the discovery of new compounds that affect these receptors may be helpful for the treatment of disorders of cognition and motivation.[19]

Direct Relevance to Psychotherapy

Although we cannot do much about the organic consequences of dementia and its affect on memory and learning, psychotherapists can be helpful and supportive with the emotional consequences of dementia, not only with the patient, but also with the family and the care-givers. We will be called upon as sources of information and support as families make decisions as to how the person with dementia is regarded and cared for as the disease progresses. Many difficult decisions arise as the patient has less and less ability to handle the tasks of daily living, such as bathing, dressing, eating, and as general care for the person with dementia becomes a full-time job for the care-giver. Families have to deal with many end-of-life issues, the need for conservatorship, power-of-attorney, "living wills," hospice care, legal and fiduciary issues as well as the many family conflicts that often arise in stressful and sad situations.

Feelings of anger, frustration, and grief are inevitable and need to be processed during the course of the disease. Although most of the therapeutic work is with families and care-givers, the therapist also has to be sensitive to the mental status of the person with dementia and his or her need for emotional and medical support, particularly in the early stages of dementia when depression is common. As therapists, it is our responsibility to be realistic and well-informed about dementia, the possible options for treatment, and the resources available so that we can best assist geriatric clients and their families.

The Alzheimer's Association, and the Center for Research on Aging, are wonderful resources for professionals and for families of patients looking for answers to questions as well as for training on issues related to dementia. All clients and their families who are coping with these disorders need to be made aware of these valuable resources.[6]

References for Chapter 10

1. Delagarza, V. W. (1998). New drugs for Alzheimer's disease. *Am. Fam. Physician,* 58(5), 1175–1182.
2. Grundman, M. & Thai, L. J. (2000). Treatment of Alzheimer's disease: Rationale and strategies. *Neurol. Clin.,* 18(4), 807–828.
3. Flint, A. J. & van Reekum, R. (1998). The pharmacologic treatment of Alzheimer's disease: A guide for the general psychiatrist. *Can. J. Psychiatry,* 43(7) 689–697.
4. Bullock, R. (2002). New drugs for Alzheimer's disease and other dementias. *Brit. J. of Psychiatry*, 180, 135–139
5. Pepeu, G., Marconcini Pepeu, I. & Amaducc, L. (1996). A review of phospho-tidylserine pharmacological and clinical effects: Is phosphotidylserine a drug for the aging brain? *Pharmacological Research*, 33,(2), 73–80.
6. Alzheimer's Association 800-272-3900. Retrieved from, http://www.alz.org/
7. Fox, N. (2000). Increased rates of atrophy in early and preclinical AD: Studies with registration of serial MRI. *Neurobiol. Aging*, 21(suppl. 1) S74, Abstract 330.
8. Fox, N., Crum, W. R., Scahill, R. & Rossor, M. N. (2001). Patterns of tissue loss in degenerative dementia detected with voxel compression mapping of serial MRI. Where does atrophy in Alzheimer's disease start and how does it progress? Program and abstracts of the 17th World Congress of Neurology; June 17–22. London, UK. *Neurol. Sci.,*187, (suppl. 1), S116. Abstract 57.05.
9. Thompson, T. L., Filley, C. M., Mitchell, W. D., Culig, K. M., Lo Verde, M. & Byyny, R. L. (1990). Lack of efficacy of Hydergine in patients with Alzheimer's disease. *New England Journal of Medicine*, 323, 445–448.
10. Van Dongen, M., Van Rossum, E., Kessels, A., Seilhorst, H. & Knipschild, P. (2000). Efficacy of ginkgo for elderly people with dementia and age-associat-ed memory impairment: New results of a randomized clinical trial. *J. American Geriatric Society*, 48, 1183–1194.
11. Singh, H. K. & Dhawan, B. N. (1982). Effect of Bacopa moniera Linn. (brahmi)

extract on avoidance response in rat. *J. Ethnopharmacol.*, 5(2), 205–214.

12. Xu, S. S., Gao, Z. X. & Weng, Z. (1999). Huperzine-A in capsules and tablets for treating patients with Alzheimer's disease. *Acta. Pharmacol. Sinica*, 20(6), 486–490.

13. Cuajungco, K. Y., Huang, X., Tanzi, R. E. & Bush, A. I. (2000). Metal chelation as a potential therapy for Alzheimer's disease. Annals of the New York Academy of Sciences, *The Molecular Basis of Dementia*, 920, 292–304.

14. Bakay, R. A., MD, Pay, M. N., RN & Merrill, D., PHD. (2002). Growth factor gene therapy for Alzheimer's disease. *Neurosurg. Focus*, 13(5), Article 5.

15. Xia, W. (2003). Amyloid inhibitors and Alzheimer's disease. *Current Opinion Investig. Drugs*, 4(1), 55–59.

16. Schenk, D., Seubert, P. & Ciccarelli, R. B. (2001). Immunotherapy with beta-amyloid for Alzheimer's disease: A new frontier. *DNA Cell Biol.*, 20(11), 679–681.

17. Johnson, S. A, Luu, N. T., Herbst, T. A., Knapp, R., Lutz, D., Arai, A., Rogers, G. A. & Lynch, G. (1999). Psychological effects of a drug that facilitates brain AMPA receptors. *J. Pharmacol. Exp. Ther.*, 289(1), 392–397.

18. Winblad, B. & Poritis, N. (1999). Memantine in severe dementia: The results of the M-Best study (Benefit and Efficacy in Severely Demented Patients During Treatment with Memantine). *International Journal of Geriatric Psychiatry*, 14, 135–136.

19. Conn, J. (2003). Glutamate and disorders of cognition and motivation. April 13–15, *New York Academy of Sciences.*

Chapter 11

Supplements, Herbs, & Oils

But flowers distill'd though they with winter meet,
Lose but their show; their substance still lives sweet.
William Shakespeare

The use of "supplements" for medicinal purposes has increased among Americans by over 400% during the last ten years.[1] No FDA approval is required for substances that are in the category of supplements. This means that they are not tested for safety and efficacy. Since these products are not regulated, we cannot even be certain that the label accurately reflects the contents of the package.

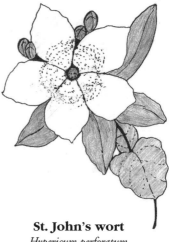

St. John's wort
Hypericum perforatum

In addition to vitamins, minerals, and other types of supplements, more than 500 "herbal products" are currently marketed in the U.S. It is estimated that approximately 60 million Americans are using these products, primarily to treat chronic physical problems, such as joint pain and high blood pressure, as well as for psychiatric disorders, in particular anxiety and depression. This chapter focuses on the preparations that are being used as sleep aids or to treat psychological symptoms.

In general, if taken one at a time and not combined with each other or with other medications, these products are considered to be safe, and many have been in use in other cultures for hundreds or even thousands of years. Data on these products' efficacy, adverse effects, safety, and interactions with other drugs has only recently begun to be collected in the U.S.

According to Tuft's Center for the Study of Drug Development, it takes between 10 and 15 years to develop and gain FDA approval to market a new prescription drug in the U.S. The average cost of this is $802 million, much of which is due to the expense of clinical trials. There is an additional cost of $95 million for testing after FDA approval, for a total cost of $897 million before a new drug can be marketed.[2] Because most of the alternative products are obtained naturally and cannot be patented, few companies that produce supplements are willing to incur this enormous expense. It is difficult for a manufacturer to commit to the huge cost of research and development if there is not potentially enough profit to be made.

Even medications approved by the FDA are sometimes found to have surprising adverse effects after they are put on the market and then taken by many thousands of people. Two well-known examples are thalidomide, which was found to cause birth defects, and various antibiotics that were later found to cause serious, and sometimes fatal, blood-disorders. This same risk exists when alternative treatments are marketed.

Before taking any medication, even FDA-approved drugs, clients need to check with their physicians and obtain as much information as possible. The longer a product has been on the market, the more that is known about its adverse effects and interactions with other compounds. The physician needs to ascertain that each drug does not interfere with any other drug taken, or worsen any medical problem. If any type of medical procedure or surgery is planned, it is particularly important for the physician to be informed of any herbal or other type of alternative medication currently being taken (including vitamins and minerals).

Vitamins, Minerals & Other Supplements

Only one person in ten eats the recommended number servings of fruits and vegetables each day, and therefore most adults do not get the Recommended Daily Allowance (RDA) of important nutrients. Many physicians advise taking a daily multivitamin/mineral supplement to make up for the nutrients that may be missing from today's typical American diet.[3]

Several minerals are known to be important for maintaining a healthy nervous system: calcium (Ca), copper (Cu), iron (Fe), phosphorus (P), potassium (K), and sodium (Na). Some (Ca, K, Na) are directly involved in the transmission of the nerve impulse down the axon. Since we need only minute amounts of each mineral, it is best to get them through one's diet. Taking mineral supplements in pill form is usually not recommended. The main exception to this is in cases where iron-deficiency anemia has been diagnosed by a physician and iron supplements are necessary.[3]

B COMPLEX VITAMINS

B vitamins are necessary for maintaining a healthy nervous system. They have a calming affect on some people and increase tolerance to stress. They should not be taken individually (unless prescribed by a physician) as this may disturb the balance of the various B vitamins to each other, causing a deficiency of one or more of the other B vitamins. Consuming alcohol, tobacco or caffeine depletes the body of vitamins and can lead to a B vitamin deficiency. Vegetarians (especially vegans) may develop a B_{12} deficiency since this vitamin is primarily present in animal products (e.g., meat, milk, cheese, eggs). B_{12} deficiency can cause symptoms of weakness and tiredness due to the disorder known as B_{12} deficiency anemia.[3]

VITAMIN E

There is some evidence that large amounts of vitamin E can slow the progression of Alzheimer's disease. This is probably due to vitamin E's antioxidant properties. When taken in high doses, vitamin E acts as an anticoagulant and lengthens the time it takes for one's blood to clot. For this reason, physicians recommend discontinuing vitamin E supplements a minimum of three weeks before any surgery.[4]

CHROMIUM PICOLINATE

A small study found that chromium picolinate, a dietary supplement, may be a safe and effective treatment for atypical depression. At the end of eight weeks, 70% of the patients on chromium improved, as opposed to 0% of the patients on placebo. Further investigation is needed to corroborate these results.[5]

DEHYDROEPIANDROSTERONE (DHEA)

In one study, the neurosteroid DHEA was added to the regular medication regimen of patients with chronic schizophrenia and prominent negative symptoms. Patients receiving the DHEA supplement had a significant reduction in their negative symptoms.[6]

OMEGA-3 FATTY ACIDS

In addition to the many reported benefits to the cardiovascular system from the use of omega-3 fatty acids, there is strong evidence to support its use for the treatment of depression. These substances are abundant in seafood, especially in oily fish like tuna, salmon, and sardines. Countries such as Japan, where fish is a mainstay of the average diet, have very low rates of both major depression and post-partum depression. There is also evidence that if omega-3 fatty acids are taken in higher doses than used for depression, there is improvement in both the manic and the depressive symptoms of bipolar disorder. The only adverse effects noted were mild GI upsets in about 25% of those treated. The mechanism of action is unknown.[7-10]

Herbal Remedies for Psychological Purposes

Herbal products have been widely used outside the U.S. for centuries, and in the past few years their use has fueled a major growth industry here. Current surveys indicate that one in three Americans has used herbal remedies. Most of these products consist of a specific part of a plant, or are made from an extract derived from part of a plant. Because some plants are composed of hundreds of different and potentially active ingredients, it is frequently difficult to determine what the active compound or compounds are, and to determine the exact amount needed for effectiveness. These factors make controlled studies of herbal remedies, where the dose of active ingredient needs to be kept constant and compared with placebo, difficult and rare.

GINKGO

Ginkgo is primarily used as a cognition-enhancing drug. It has been

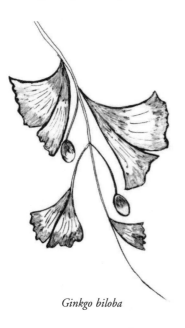

Ginkgo biloba

evaluated for this use in Alzheimer's disease, and most studies show that there is cognitive improvement if ginkgo is taken for three to twelve months. Some people show improvement after only one month of treatment. The improvement has been evaluated using objective tests for cognition. It is thought that ginkgo exerts its effect by its ability to dilate blood vessels, and that cognition is improved because the blood supply throughout the brain increases. However, a recent placebo-controlled study showed no meaningful measurable effect (see page 149).[11]

Adverse effects of ginkgo

There are few adverse effects. Most frequently seen are:

- headache
- sensitivity to light
- gastrointestinal problems

Ginkgo inhibits platelet aggregation, resulting in an increase in clotting time and an increased risk of excessive bleeding. For this reason, it is not recommended that ginkgo be used concurrently with anticoagulants. Due to the increased risk of hemorrhage, people with diabetes and hypertension should avoid ginkgo. Its use may increase the frequency of headaches in people who suffer from migraines.[12]

GINSENG

Ginseng (*Panax ginseng*) and Siberian ginseng (*Eleutherococcus senticosus*) are believed to improve mood, enhance energy, and reduce stress. Studies have been done comparing ginseng to placebo and to a multivitamin, with contradictory findings. This may be due to the variability of the active ingredient in different ginseng preparations. In addition, at least 20 different ginsenosides (ginseng alkaloids) have been identified; each may have different pharmacological activity, and some of the activities may oppose each other.

Adverse effects of ginseng

- corticosteroid-like activity
- a decrease in blood glucose
- inhibition of platelet aggregation
- estrogenic effect (generates estrogen)
- can produce vaginal bleeding and swollen breasts

There is one case report of a negative result due to the interaction of ginseng and phenelzine, an MAO inhibitor. A depressed patient experienced mania, insomnia, and headache after taking ginseng and phenelzine.[13]

KAVA

Kava *(Piper methysticum)* is used mainly for reduction of anxiety and as a sleep-inducing agent. Several controlled studies using objective measures for anxiety have found kava to be effective in reducing anxiety. Positive effects were seen as early as one week after treatment. Recently, a meta-analysis has been done which validates that kava is superior to placebo in all of the reviewed trials. It is believed that kava works by blocking NE reuptake, suppressing the release of glutamate, and increasing GABA receptor density.[14]

Adverse effects of kava

Very few of the patients studied in the U.S. complained of any adverse effects with kava. There were a few complaints of:

- restlessness • mild GI upset • tremor

It is believed that ingredients in kava act as skeletal muscle relaxants and as anticonvulsants. A comatose state was reported in a patient who took kava and was already taking alprazolam/Xanax (a BZ), cimetadine, and terazosin. The coma occurred three days after taking kava. The use of multiple drugs made the interpretation of the interactions inconclusive. The patient recovered without significant problems.[14, 15] Twenty-five cases of liver toxicity that occurred in Switzerland and Germany have been reported to the FDA. It is unclear whether the toxicity was due to kava or to other factors.

ST. JOHN'S WORT (SJW)

St. John's wort *(Hypericum perforatum)* is believed to block reuptake of NE and 5-HT. It has been used for many years as an antidepressant in Germany, where clinical trials have indicated efficacy comparable to TCAs. SJW has recently gained popularity in the United States. There have been many recent studies comparing the efficacy of SJW to placebo or TCAs; most show SJW to be effective in treating mild to moderate depressions.[16] However, one recent, carefully-controlled study found that the effectiveness of taking SJW was not significantly greater than taking a placebo.[17]

Treatment of somatoform disorders with SJW

Research indicates that SJW is effective for the treatment of somatoform disorders independent of depressed mood. The researchers conclude that the specific advantages of SJW are safety, absence of sedating effect, and fast treatment onset.[18]

Adverse effects of SJW

The most frequently seen adverse effects are mild GI symptoms and fatigue. People with epilepsy should consult their physicians before taking SJW, since there have been reports of an increase in seizure activity when taking the drug. SJW may increase the frequency and duration of migraine headaches. Photosensitivity has been reported in light-sensitive people taking high doses of SJW. This effect was reversed when SJW was discontinued. Excessive sedation was reported in one elderly subject who was also taking paroxetine. Symptoms included lethargy, slow response time, and limp muscle tone. It is recommended that SJW not be used in conjunction with MAO inhibitors or with foods containing tyramine (see p. 52).

Since SJW is reported to interact with a number of other medications, it is advisable to use caution when it is taken in combination with any other compound. This is particularly relevant for drugs that may have a stimulating effect such as:

- caffeine
- any antidepressants
- disulfiram/Antabuse
- immunosuppressive drugs
- theophylline (an asthma medication)
- over-the-counter cough and cold medicines
- any other herbal products[16]

WARNING: There is evidence that taking St. John's wort decreases the effectiveness of birth control pills.

S-ADENOSYLMETHIONINE (SAM-E)

SAM-e was isolated in 1952 and has been found to be present in all living cells. It is now being referred to as a "nutraceutical," a natural product that promotes good health and well-being. SAM-e is formed from the combination of adenosine triphosphate/ATP and the amino acid methionine. It is thought to enhance DA and 5-HT metabolism, and to repair the myelin which surrounds some nerve cells.

SAM-e is being used to treat depression. A meta-analysis was done of over 1,000 patients that suggests that SAM-e was 17% to 38% better than placebo, and elicited a faster response than the antidepressant drug imipramine/Tofranil.[19]

Cautions on the use of SAM-e
- It should not be taken along with other antidepressants.
- It can induce a manic episode in people with bipolar disorder.
- It may decrease fertility in women.
- The active ingredients in SAM-e tend to break down rapidly, so the dose indicated on the label may not accurately reflect the contents of the tablets.[20]

VALERIAN

This herb *(Valeriana officinalis)* works immediately to reduce feelings of nervousness, and to improve the quality of sleep, by decreasing both sleep latency and nocturnal awakenings due to anxiety. It is believed to exert its effect through interaction with GABA receptors.[21]

Adverse effects of valerian
Valerian causes drowsiness; one should not drive or operate dangerous machinery after taking it. Some people have a drug hangover in the morning after taking it to help with sleep. Valerian should not be used while taking any other sleep or antianxiety medications.[22]

Essential Oils (Aromatherapy)

This section is intended to be used as a quick-reference guide for the psychotherapist who has clients who are using aromatherapy. There are many books on aromatherapy, and clients need to thoroughly educate themselves in the appropriate uses of, and the dangers associated with, each oil.

Aromatherapy practitioners often describe their practice as the art of healing with the concentrated extracts from plants, herbs, and flowers that are called "essential oils." They are said to be able to relieve stress, depression, and mental fatigue as well as a variety of physical ailments. Aromatherapy is growing by proverbial leaps and bounds, but how (or if) it works is yet to be scientifically proven.[23]

Route of administration

The sense of smell is believed to be the most evocative of all the senses. The theoretical basis for the effectiveness of aromatherapy is that a connection exists between the sense of smell and the brain which can promote relaxation, increase energy, and restore balance to the mind. Aromatherapists believe that these scents work by influencing the limbic area of the brain to balance the nervous system and calm the emotions. Practitioners claim that aromatherapy bolsters the individual's ability to cope with stress.[24]

All of these oils can be diluted in water and used as room misters. Putting a few drops of oil in a glass of water for misting is enough to get a pleasant scent. A few drops can be put on a tissue to carry and inhale throughout the day, or placed on a pillow at bedtime.[25]

Adverse reactions to essential oils

Some essential oils irritate the eyes and other mucous membranes, and are not to be applied directly to the skin without being diluted. A patch test for allergy is generally recommended before using any of these oils.[24-26]

Essential Oils & Their Uses for Psychological Purposes

Bergamot – treats depression, relieves anxiety

Blue Tansy – reduces stress, increases feelings of well-being

Celery – sedates

Chamomile – calms, reduces stress, irritability & depression

Citrus – relaxes and calms

Clary Sage – helps with symptoms of PMS, relaxes muscles, calms

Clove – treats symptoms of fatigue

Geranium – sedates, treats nervousness

Lavender – reduces headaches, relieves insomnia, reduces symptoms of PMS, reduces stress

Lemon grass – calms

Marjoram – calms, warms, soothes

Melaleuca – calms jangled nerves, relieves pain

Melissa – treats depression

Mint – clears the mind

Neroli – treats depression & anxiety

Orange – lifts spirits

Patchouli – relaxes

Pennyroyal – stimulates

Peppermint – improves mental acuity, decreases fatigue

Rose – calms nerves, assuages anger

Rosemary – clears the mind, energizes, helps memory

Rosewood – clears the head

Sage – relaxes

Sandalwood – calms nerves, relieves anxiety

Tangerine – lifts spirits

Thyme – stimulates the brain

Turkish rose – stimulates, elevates the mind

Wintergreen – stimulates

Ylang ylang – relieves tension, soothes, helps with PMS

Ylang ylang
Cananga odorata

From *Drugs & Clients, What Every Psychotherapist Needs to Know* by Padma Catell. © 2004   Table 11.1

WARNING: These oils are not to be taken internally. If irritation develops the use of the oil should be discontinued immediately.

Direct Relevance to Psychotherapy

All of the substances discussed in this chapter can be obtained with relative ease. Most people consider these to be safe for self-medication, and many clients do not think of them as "drugs" and therefore do not mention taking them to their psychotherapist or their psychiatrist. As the use of these products grows, the incidence of adverse effects and interactions with other drugs will also increase. It is important that the psychotherapist ask if the client is using any herbal or "alternative" products (supplements, vitamins, or minerals) in addition to any prescription or illicit drugs.

The herbs and other products discussed here are medicinal agents and have a psychoactive effect. The psychotherapist needs to caution clients about possible drug interactions. The therapist may be the first person to observe any overdose or adverse effect from these products. The FDA now maintains a database on adverse effects associated with herbal use that can be accessed at http://vm.cfsan.fda.gov/.

References for Chapter 11

1. Fugh-Berman, A. (2000). Herb-drug interactions. *Lancet*, 355, 134–138.
2. Tuft's Center for the Study of Development. Retrieved Aug. 31, 2003 from http://csdd.tufts.edu/NewsEvents/recentNews.asp?newsid=6
3. Turnland, J. R. (1994). Future directions for establishing mineral/trace element requirements. *J. Nutr.*, 124(9 suppl.), 1765S–1770S.
4. Bullock, R. (2002). New drugs for Alzheimer's disease and other dementias. *Brit. J. of Psychiatry*, 180, 135–139
5. Davidson, J. R. T., Abraham, K., Connor, M. N. & McLeod, M. N. (2003). Effectiveness of chromium in atypical depression: A placebo-controlled trial. *Biological psychiatry*, 53(3), 261–264.
6. Rabkin, J. G., Ferrando, S. J., Wagner, G. J. & Rabkin, R. (2000). DHEA treatment for HIV+ patients: Effects on mood, androgenic and anabolic parameters. *Psychoneuroendocrin.*, Jan., 25(1), 53–68.
7. Hibbeln, J. R. (1998). Fish consumption and major depression. *Lancet*, 351(9110), 1213.
8. Stoll, A. L. (1999). Omega-3 fatty acids in bipolar disorder: A preliminary, double blind, placebo controlled trial. *Arch. Gen. Psych.*, 56(5), 407–412.
9. Calabrese, J. R., Rapport, D. J. & Shelton, M. D. (1999). Fish oils and bipolar disorder: A promising but untested treatment. *Arch. Gen. Psychiatry*, 56, 413–416.

10. Zanarini, M. & Frankenburg, F. (2003). Omega-3 fatty-acid treatment of women with borderline personality disorder: A double-blind, placebo-controlled pilot study. *Am. J. of Psychiatry*, 160, 167–169.

11. Van Dongen, M., Van Rossum, E., Kessels, A., Seilhorst, H. & Knipschild, P. (2000). Efficacy of ginkgo for elderly people with dementia and age-associated memory impairment: New results of a randomized clinical trial. *J. American Geriatric Society*, 48, 1183–1194.

12. Vale, S. (1998). Subarachnoid hemorrhage associated with ginkgo biloba. *Lancet*, 352–356.

13. Jones, B. D. & Runikis, A. M. (1987). Interaction of ginseng with phenelizine. *J. Clinical Psychopharm.*, 7, 201–202.

14. Pittler, M. H. & Ernst, E. (2000). Efficacy of kava extract for treating anxiety: Systemic review and meta-analysis. *J. Clinical Psychopharm.*, 20, 84–89.

15. Almeida, J. C. & Grimsley, E. W. (1996). Coma from the health food store: Interaction between kava and alprazolam. *Annals of Internal Medicine*, 125, 940–941.

16. Linde, K., Ramirez, G., Mulrow, C. D., Pauls, A., Weidenhammer, W. & Melchart, D. (1996). St. John's wort for depression: An overview and meta-analysis of randomized clinical trials. *British Medical Journal*, 313, 253–258.

17. Shelton, R. C., Keller, M. B., Gelenberg, A., Dunner, D. L., Hirschfeld, R., Thase, M. E., Russell, J., Lydiard, R. B., Crits-Cristoph, P., Gallop, R., Todd, L., Hellerstein, D., Goodnick, P., Keitner, G., Stahl, S. M., & Halbreich, U. (2001). Effectiveness of St. John's Wort in major depression: A randomized clinical trial. *JAMA*, 285(15), 1978–1986.

18. Voltz, H. P., Murck, H., Kaspar, S. & Moller, H. J. (2002). St. John's Wort extract (LI 160) in somatoform disorders: Results of a placebo controlled trial. *Psychopharmacology*, 164, 294–300.

19. Chiaie, R. & Pancheri, P. (2002). Efficacy and tolerability of oral and intramuscular S-adenosyl-L-methionine 1,4-butanedisulfonate (SAMe) in the treatment of major depression: Comparison with imipramine in 2 multicenter studies. *Am. J. Clin. Nutr.*, 76(suppl.), 1172S–1176S.

20. Bottiglieri, T. (1997). Ademetionine (S-adenosylmethionine) neuropharmacology: Implications for drug therapies in psychiatric and neurological disorders. *Expert Opinion in Investigational Drugs*, 6, 417–426.

21. Donath, F., Quispe, K., Maurer, A., Fietze, I. & Roots, I. (2000). Critical Evaluation of the effect of valerian extract on sleep structure and sleep quality. *Pharmacopsychiatry*, 33, 47–53.

22. Santillo, H. (1984). *Natural healing with herbs*. Prescott Valley, Arizona: HOHM Press.

23. Dunn, C., Sleep, J. & Collett, D. (1995). Sensing an improvement: An experimental study to evaluate the use of aromatherapy, massage, and periods of rest in an intensive care unit. *J. Adv. Nursing*, 21, 34–40.

24. Green, M. & Keville, K. (1995). *Aromatherapy a complete guide to the healing art*. Santa Cruz, CA: Crossing Press.

25. Rose, J. (1992). *The aromatherapy book: Applications and inhalations*. Berkeley, CA: North Atlantic Books.

26. Jackson, M. & Teague, T. (1975). *The handbook of alternatives to chemical medicine*. Berkeley, CA: Lawton-Teague Publications.

Appendix A

The Nerve Cell & the Brain

This section is intended to provide psychotherapists, whose training typically does not include advanced courses in biochemistry and anatomy, with a simplified frame of reference to the underpinnings of the beliefs and concepts that shape modern psychopharmacology. It is the specific purview and responsibility of psychiatrists, who do have specific training and a thorough understanding of neurochemistry and the mechanisms of action for the psychoactive drugs, to determine which is best for each individual patient.

Structure of the Nerve Cell

Pharmacological treatment of psychological problems is based on the current understanding of the biochemical processes in the central nervous system (CNS), in particular, the use of drugs that influence neuromodulators, neurotransmitters, and other substances that affect nerve cells. These medications target various parts of the transmitter system to cause changes in the processes in the CNS. These changes ultimately affect cognition, emotions, and behavior.

The nerve cell (neuron) is the basic unit of the nervous system (See Figures A1, The Neuron, p. 170, and C1, The Synapse, p. 179). The parts and components of the nerve cell are:

Axon: This is the structure along which nerve impulses are transmitted to presynaptic terminals. (See Fig. A1.)

COMT: Catechol-O-methyltransferase is an enzyme present in the synaptic cleft. (See Fig. C1.)

Dendrites: These are branching structures that receive impulses from adjacent nerve cells. (See Fig. C1.)

MAO: Monoamine oxidase is an enzyme present in the presynaptic terminal. (See Fig. C1.)

Myelin sheath: This covers the axon in some nerve cells. (See Fig. A1.)

Nodes of Ranvier : These are pores in the myelin sheath that allow the impulse to "jump" along the axon from one node to the next by a process called "saltation." It is at these nodes where charged particles (ions) pass through the cell membrane, allowing the impulse to travel down the axon very rapidly as the cell depolarizes.[1] (See Fig. A1.)

Presynaptic terminal: This structure contains the synaptic vesicles. (See Fig. C1.)

Soma (or cell body): This contains the nucleus and organelles that synthesize and package protein (e.g., Golgi apparatus, endoplasmic reticulum, mitochondria). (See Fig. A1.)

Synaptic cleft: The space between nerve cells where transmitter substances make contact with receptors. (See Fig. C1.)

Synaptic vesicles: Sites where transmitter substances are stored and protected from enzymatic degradation by monoamine oxidase (MAO). (See Fig. C1.)

The Neuron

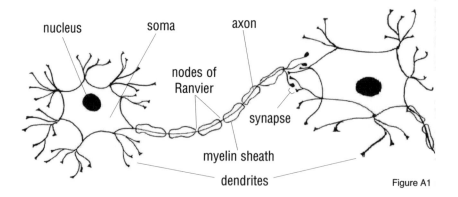

Figure A1

Glial Cells

Glial cells (see Fig. B1, p. 174) are another type of cell found in the nervous system. These cells function as structural support and nutrition for neurons. They also produce myelin, and are an important component of the blood-brain barrier. Glial cells are now known to also have receptors for transmitters.[2]

The "white matter" in the brain is composed of nerve fibers coated with myelin; "gray matter" is composed of nerve fibers that are not coated with myelin. The myelin forms a fatty sheath around the nerve fiber which makes it appear white.[1]

Transmission of the Nerve Impulse

When a nerve cell is in a "resting" state, the concentration of sodium ions (Na^{+1}) is high extracellularly (outside the cell), and low intracellularly (inside the cell). Potassium (K^{+1}) has the opposite concentration (low outside, high inside). Chlorine (Cl^{-1}) is largely extracellular, and its charge is balanced by negatively charged amino acids and proteins inside the cell. Positively charged calcium ions (Ca^{+2}) exist in free form in the cytoplasm, and these have a major role in control of many cellular functions (e.g., the activation of enzymes, and the release of compounds from synaptic vesicles). Most

Distribution of Ions

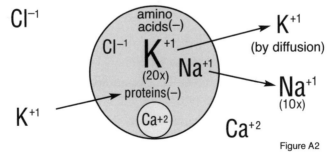

Figure A2

intracellular Ca^{+2} is sequestered in organelles, such as the endoplasmic reticulum and mitochondria, which keeps the concentration of free Ca^{+2} very low. When the concentration of free Ca^{+2} rises, the processes that are dependent on free Ca^{+2} are initiated.[1]

Unequal distribution of ions across cell membranes results in a "resting membrane potential" (the interior of the cell is negatively charged relative to its exterior). Neuronal firing requires a change in this resting potential. A decrease in potential leads to depolarization. The interior of the cell becomes less negative with respect to the extracellular space; this makes the cell more likely to fire, therefore it is considered "excitatory." An increase in potential (i.e., the interior of the cell becomes even more negatively charged) is termed "hyperpolarization." This process makes the cell less likely to fire, and is therefore termed "inhibitory."[1]

One way a nerve cell's membrane potential is regulated is through ion channels. These channels consist of glycoprotein molecules that traverse the membrane. Changes in the structure of these protein molecules cause an opening and closing of pores through which certain ions can pass. Unique properties of these glycoproteins allow for selection of ions and specific circumstances under which the channel will open. The open state of the channel has a specific time-course and conductance. A channel may have more than one "open" state (time-course and conductance can differ for the same channel).

Certain channels, called "ligand-gated channels," are closely linked to receptors and open when the neurotransmitter or neuromodulator binds to the receptor. Other channels, designated "voltage-gated channels," respond to the degree of membrane polarization.[1]

Specific inhibitory or excitatory neurotransmitters bind to receptor molecules. A transmitter substance, depending on the location within the brain, can be both excitatory *and* inhibitory. The binding leads to a change in ion conductance, or to the activation of a "second messenger" within the cell, the transmitter substance itself being the "first messenger." Activation of the second messenger system can have several effects, including the activation of enzymes that manufacture neuronal proteins, an alteration of membrane conductance, or a change in rate of protein synthesis.[3]

Summary

Transmission of the nerve impulse is an electro-chemical phenomenon. The cell is depolarized by a flow of ions from one side of the membrane to the other, generating a charge or current that then passes down the axon. When the impulse arrives at the nerve cell terminal, it stimulates release of substances from synaptic vesicles. Transmitter substances are then released into the synaptic cleft (separation between nerve cells), where transmitters contact receptors on the cell membrane of the dendrites of the next nerve cell.

There are many examples where neurons release transmitters in regions that lack the specialization of the classical nerve synapse. Nevertheless, the simplified concept described here, that a transmitter released from a presynaptic cell contacts a postsynaptic receptor which then recognizes the transmitter and responds, remains useful to an understanding of most nerve-cell functions.[1]

The interaction of a specific transmitter with a receptor will lead to either depolarization (firing) or to hyperpolarization (inhibition) of the next nerve cell. It is important to realize that at any one time each nerve cell is receiving input from many (probably hundreds) of adjacent nerve cells. The nerve cell essentially "sums up" all of the information it is receiving, and depending upon the net result of the summation, the next neuron will either fire or be inhibited.

References for Appendix A

1. Hyman, S. E., MD. (1988). Recent developments in neurobiology: Part 1. synaptic transmission. *Psychosomatics*, 29(2).
2. Bloom, F. E. & Kupfer, D. J. (Eds.). (1995). *Psychopharmacology: The fourth generation of progress.* New York: Raven Press.
3. Julian, Robert, MD, PhD. (1995). *A primer of drug action* (7th ed.). New York: W. H. Freeman & Co.

Appendix B
Studying the Brain

There are many obstacles to doing research on the CNS. The first and most obvious one is that the brain is enclosed in the skull, making physical access to CNS neurons very difficult. The second major obstacle is the filtering system known as the blood-brain barrier.

The Blood-Brain Barrier

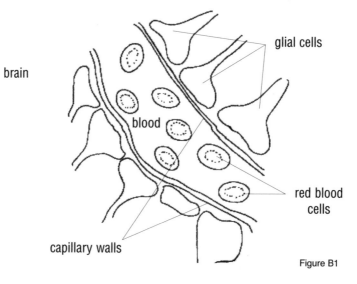

brain

glial cells

blood

red blood cells

capillary walls

Figure B1

Studying metabolism in the organs outside the brain is possible by simply obtaining a sample of blood from a vein, usually in the arm. One can be relatively certain that the blood sample is representative of venous blood throughout the body. The blood's chemical profile can be analyzed and accurate deductions made regarding metabolic processes taking place in various organs (e.g., liver, kidney). Unfortunately, this method does not work to obtain information about metabolism inside the brain, which is protected by the blood-brain barrier from many chemicals and compounds. This barrier is made up of capillaries that are packed tightly together and covered by a fatty sheath. This sheath is produced by the astrocyte type of glial cell.[1] (Figure B1.)

All the blood that enters and leaves the brain must pass through this filter. The pores in the capillaries are very small, making it difficult for large molecules to enter the brain, and the fatty makeup of the sheath makes it difficult for water-soluble molecules to get through. Therefore, a blood sample taken from the arm does not have the same chemical composition as blood in the brain. The blood-brain barrier protects the brain but makes studying the brain biochemistry and metabolism very difficult.

SCANNING TECHNIQUES

Technological advances such as MRI and PET scans are facilitating exploration and understanding of brain metabolism. An American chemist and a British physicist, Paul C. Lauterbur and Peter Mansfield, were awarded the 2003 Nobel Prize for their work in the early 1970's that resulted in the development of MRI technology, which has led the way to numerous medical advances.[2]

Magnetic resonance imaging (MRI)

This technique is possible because the water atoms in the body can be lined up with magnets and moved with radio signals. First, all the water molecules in the body are lined up in a North-South direction. A radio signal then is used to move the water molecules away from their North-South orientation. The energy required to move the molecules varies depending upon the density of the structures in the body. This variance is analyzed and converted to digital images that represent anatomy.[3]

The Limbic System

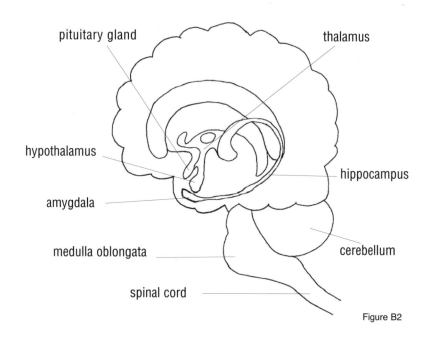

pituitary gland

thalamus

hypothalamus

hippocampus

amygdala

medulla oblongata

cerebellum

spinal cord

Figure B2

Positron emission tomography (PET)

PET scans facilitate the comparison of the degree of metabolic activity between different areas of the brain and the tracking of metabolic changes over time. This is useful for observing changes that occur in the progression of a disease, the influences of various psychoactive medications on the brain, and changes in a subject's brain activity while looking at or thinking about different things. PET scans also enable comparisons of brain activity between people who have been diagnosed with a mental disorder, and those who have not.

PET and MRI scans are being refined to yield more detailed and specific information. With these new techniques it is becoming possible to label, localize, and map various neurotransmitters and neuromodulators, to study how they function, and to observe the progression of diseases such as Parkinson's and Alzheimer's.

Prior to the development of scanning techniques like MRI and PET, mapping was done on brain slices after autopsy, and could not reflect what was occurring in the brain of a living person. The current explosion in central nervous system research and understanding is largely due to development of new instruments for neuroimaging, such as PET and fMRI (functional MRI) scanners.[4,5]

It is important to remember that microscopic techniques for clarifying the details of what occurs at the synapse have not yet been developed, so information about CNS activity at the synaptic level is still very theoretical.

References for Appendix B

1. Julian, Robert, MD, PhD. (1995). *A primer of drug action* (7th ed.). New York: W. H. Freeman & Co.
2. Pincock, S. (2003) MRI scientists win Nobel Prize: Lauterbur and Mansfield lauded for contribution to imaging technique. *The Scientist.* Oct. 6. Retrieved Oct. 18, 2003 from http://www.biomedcentral.com/news/20031006/06
3. Shalen, P. R., MD. (2002). MRI. Retrieved Oct. 19, 2003 from http://www.spine-health.com/topics/diag/mri/mri_scan02.html
4. Fox, N. (2000). Increased rates of atrophy in early and preclinical AD: Studies with registration of serial MRI. *Neurobiol. Aging,* 21(suppl. 1), S74. Abstract 330.
5. Fox, N., Crum, W. R., Scahill, R. & Rossor, M. N. (2001). Patterns of tissue loss in degenerative dementia detected with voxel compression mapping of serial MRI. Where does atrophy in Alzheimer's disease start and how does it progress? Program and abstracts of the 17th World Congress of Neurology; June 17–22; London, UK. J *Neurol. Sci.,* 187(suppl. 1), S116. Abstract 57.05.

Appendix C
Transmitter Substances

Transmitter substances are usually small molecules that relay information from the end of one nerve cell across the synaptic cleft to the receptor of the next nerve cell. The nomenclature is changing, and some substances that were previously called "neurotransmitters" are now being called "neuromodulators."

A neuromodulator is a chemical that modulates neuronal transmission that is primarily facilitated by some other neurotransmitter. A neuromodulator can make receptors either more or less sensitive to a neurotransmitter. Norepinephrine (NE), dopamine (DA), and serotonin (5-HT) are now considered neuromodulators to the amino acid neurotransmitters (primarily GABA and glutamate).[1-3]

Central Nervous System Transmitter Substances

ACETYLCHOLINE (ACH)

Acetylcholine (ACh) was the first neurotransmitter to be identified. It was initially found in the peripheral nervous system (PNS), where it is the major neurotransmitter at the neuromuscular junction. ACh is also present in large amounts in the brain, with the highest concentrations found in the cerebral cortex and the caudate nucleus.[4] ACh is also present in the basal ganglia, where it plays a role in the mediation of movement. When the balance between ACh and DA is disturbed, various movement disorders occur. Examples of this are the extrapyramidal syndrome (EPS) sometimes seen with antipsychotic medications, and the problems with movement seen with Parkinson's disease. ACh is involved in other processes such as:

- mood
- learning
- memory
- attention
- REM sleep
- behavioral arousal

ACh is involved in Alzheimer's disease, and in the negative symptoms of schizophrenia.[5]

The Synapse

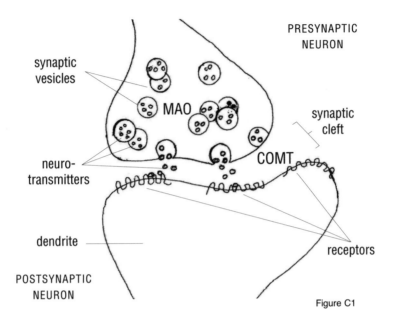

Figure C1

AMINO ACID TRANSMITTERS

Amino acids are very abundant as neurotransmitters in the brain, and can be found at about 90% of CNS transmitting sites.[6] Neurons also use amino acids to make proteins and other neurotransmitters. Some amino acids (e.g., glutamate and aspartate) are excitatory, while others (e.g., GABA and glycine) are inhibitory.[7]

Aspartate & glutamate

The amino acids aspartate and glutamate are the main excitatory transmitters in the CNS. Glutamate is replacing dopamine as the current focus of psychopharmacology research. Drugs that act on the glutamate transporter are being tested for the treatment of anxiety disorders, schizophrenia, and addiction.[2]

Gamma-aminobutyric acid (GABA)

GABA, which is thought to be the main inhibitory amino acid transmitter in the CNS, has been investigated quite extensively. Much of the research has been done on the role of GABA receptors in the action of the BZs.[8] Neurons that use GABA as their transmitting agent function primarily as interneurons in many areas of the brain. Two types of GABA receptors are GABA/A and GABA/B. In the brain, GABA/A receptors are directly coupled to chloride ion channels. After activation by GABA/A, the channel becomes permeable to chloride ions, and the neuron becomes hyperpolarized (inhibited). This inhibition seems to lead to a decrease in neuronal activity and a decrease in anxiety.[9]

MONOAMINE TRANSMITTERS (DA, NE, 5-HT)

Though less abundant than the amino acid transmitters, these substances are very potent in their activity. The monoamines are thought to mainly modulate or "fine tune" the actions of the amino acid NTs, GABA, and glutamate.[1-3] It is known that each monoamine transmitter has many subtypes that seem to affect different processes and areas of the CNS.

Dopamine (DA)

Large amounts of dopamine can be found in the nerve cells that terminate in the basal ganglia, frontal cortex, and limbic system. These nerve cells have their cell bodies in the substantia nigra of the brain stem and in the limbic system (Fig. B2). There is evidence that DA can be both excitatory and inhibitory.[1] DA has a role in:

- emotional reactions
- thought processes
- schizophrenia
- addictions
- normal movement
- Parkinson's disease

It is not yet possible for a drug to target only one part of the brain, so all of these functions are affected to some degree by drugs that act on dopaminergic synapses. It is likely that the catatonic symptoms seen in some schizophrenic patients, such as muscle stiffness, bizarre positions, and loss of spontaneous movement, are also due to disturbances in the dopamine system.[2]

Norepinephrine (NE)

Areas of the brain where NE is found include the brain stem, cerebral cortex, limbic system, hypothalamus, cerebellum, and dorsal horn of the spinal cord. Processes that NE seems to influence include:

- state of arousal
- depressive disorders
- attention
- concentration
- regulation of blood pressure[6,7,10]
- analgesia
- mania
- memory
- socialization

Serotonin (5-HT)

5-HT is found mainly in the brain stem and in the neurons of the reticular formation. These reticular neurons project to many other areas of the brain. 5-HT is also found in the cortex, the hypothalamus, the hippocampus, and the limbic system (Fig. C2). 5-HT usually acts as an inhibitory neuromodulator. It has been shown to have a role in the processes of:

- depression
- sexual activity
- falling asleep
- regulating body temperature

In the depressive disorders, 5-HT is thought to affect appetite, irritability, and impulse control.[6,7,10]

NEUROPEPTIDE TRANSMITTERS

The number of neuropeptide transmitter substances exceeds the number of transmitters in all other categories. These peptides are found in some neurons that use amino acids, and in some that use amines as neurotransmitters. In these neurons, there may be a release of two or more different transmitter substances, which would allow for transmission of more complex signals to adjacent neurons. Some peptides that augment other substances act as neuromodulators.[7] Some neuropeptides that have been extensively investigated are vasopressin and oxytocin (both affect learning and memory), Substance P (involved in transmission of painful stimuli), and opioid neuropeptides (involved in analgesic responses).[11]

Hypocretin (orexin)

This substance may be responsible for preventing the spontaneous periods of REM sleep as occurs in narcolepsy. This neurotransmitter is low in humans with narcolepsy, and missing entirely in the dogs used to study this disorder in the laboratory.[12]

Opioid neuropeptides

Many areas of the central nervous system have high concentrations of specialized receptors called opioid receptors. These areas are the brain stem, medial thalamus, spinal cord, and limbic system, specifically the amygdala. Most of these areas are involved with the pain response. Some opioid receptors in the brain stem affect feelings of nausea and vomiting, while others regulate blood pressure, stomach secretions, and the cough-response. The opioid-rich areas in the limbic system mediate emotional responses.[11]

Substance P (neurokinin, NK)

Substance P, which is often abbreviated NK (neurokinin), is a member of a group of neuropeptides called "tachykinins." Its receptor is called NK1. The role of NK is as a modulator, which signals the intensity of noxious or aversive stimuli (nociception). Evidence suggests that this neuropeptide is an integral part of central nervous system pathways involved in psychological stress.[11]

NK neurons are unique in that they have receptors all over the cell body. NK is found in both the brain and spinal cord. When an area is inflamed, both the amount of NK and the number of NK receptors increase. In the brain NK receptors are found primarily in the limbic system, including two areas associated with emotional behavior, the hypothalamus and the amygdala. Approximately 10% of all neurons in the amygdala are NK neurons. Stimulation of these neurons produces anxiety. The highest density of NK neurons is in the area of the thalamus known as the habenula.[11]

NK and NK1 are present in neurons that are involved in the integration of pain, stress, and anxiety. NK1 is highly expressed in the hypothalamus, the pituitary, and the amygdala, brain regions that are critical for the regulation of emotions and neurochemical responses to stress. Also associated with the amygdala are neural pathways that respond to stressors, such as noxious or aversive stimuli.[11]

So far, using NK antagonists to decrease pain has not been successful. The use of NK antagonists for treating anxiety disorders and for the control of vomiting looks promising.

NEUROSTEROIDS

Other molecules that have properties as transmitters are the neurosteroids. Some neurosteroids are synthesized in the central nervous system and have a role in regulation of glial cells.[7]

NUCLEOTIDES

Nucleotides, such as adenosine triphosphate (ATP), sensitize neurons and enhance the response to either amine or amino acid neurotransmitters. These compounds are sometimes called "3rd messengers." [9]

Storage & Release of Monoamine Transmitters

NE, DA, and 5-HT are stored in synaptic vesicles; their release from vesicles is a calcium-dependent phenomenon. For release to take place after a nerve is stimulated, calcium must be present in the extracellular space. The release is dependent upon an influx of calcium ions (Ca^{+2}) into the nerve terminal.[4] Medications known as "calcium channel blockers" inhibit Ca^{+2} influx and block neuronal firing. This prevents stimulation of the next neuron.[7]

Some mechanism must exist to terminate the action of these substances. This can happen various ways:

After release, NE, DA, and 5-HT can be metabolized to inactive compounds by the enzyme which is present in the synapse, catechol-O-methyl transferase (COMT).

Transmitter substances may be taken back into pre-synaptic nerve terminals (reuptake), or inactivated by the enzyme monoamine oxidase (MAO).

After reuptake, they can be taken back into synaptic vesicles and stored for release at a later time.

When inside the synaptic vesicles, these substances are protected from enzymatic degradation.[4]

References for Appendix C

1. Gladwell, S. J. & Coote, J. H. (1999). Inhibitory and indirect excitatory effects of dopamine on sympathetic preganglionic neurons in the neonatal rat spinal cord in vitro. *Brain Research*, 818, 397–407.
2. Holden, C. (2003). Excited by glutamate. *Science,* 20 June, (300), 1866–1868.
3. Gainetdinov, R. R., Wetsel, W. C., Jones, S. R., Levin, E. D., Jaber, & M., Caron, M. G. R. (1999). Role of serotonin in the paradoxical calming effect of psychostimulants on hyperactivity. *Science,* 283(5400), 397–401.
4. Julian, Robert, MD, PHD. (1995). *A primer of drug action* (7th ed.). New York: W. H. Freeman & Co.
5. Grundman, M. & Thai, L. J. (2000). Treatment of Alzheimer's disease: Rationale and strategies. *Neurol. Clin.,* 18(4), 807–828.
6. Cooper, J. R., Bloom, F. E. & Roth R. H. (1995) *The biochemical basis of neuropharmacology* (7 ed.). Oxford University Press.
7. Bloom, F. E., Kupfer, D. J. (Eds.). (1995). *Psychopharmacology: The fourth generation of progress.* New York: Raven Press.
8. Haefely, W. (1990). Benzodiazepine receptor and ligands: Structural and functional differences. In: I. Hindmarch, G. Beaumont, S. Brandon, B. E. Leonard (Eds.), Benzodiazepines: Current concepts. pp. 1–18, New York: Wiley.
9. Johansen, Chris-Ellyn. (1992). *Psychopharmacology: Basic mechanisms and applied*

interventions. Washington, DC: APA.

10. Dement, W. C. & Vaughan, C. (1999). *The promise of sleep: A pioneer in sleep medicine explores the vital connection between health, happiness, and a good night's sleep.* New York, NY: Delacorte Press.

11. DeVane, C. L., Pharm.D. (2001). Substance P: A new era, a new role. *Pharmacotherapy,* 21(9), 1061–1069.

12. Hungs, M. & Mignot, E. (2001). Hypocretin/orexin, sleep and narcolepsy. *Bioessays,* 23, 397–408.

Appendix D

Proposed Mechanisms of Action

As the workings of the central nervous system are better understood, the theories explaining the mechanisms of actions of the many drugs studied in psychopharmacology become more and more complex. The techniques and technologies required to investigate details of these processes in the CNS, and at the synapse in particular, are not yet available. For this reason, the specific, detailed mechanisms of action for most psychoactive substances is not yet completely clear, and their effects are not fully understood.

Even when the primary effect of a drug is clear, this knowledge may not explain how the drug acts to create changes in emotions and behavior. This Appendix presents proposed mechanisms of action for some of the drugs included in this book. The theories as to these mechanisms of action are constantly being refined and changed as new discoveries are made.

It is known that most psychoactive substances will ultimately affect the synthesis, storage, release, reuptake, or metabolism of the neuromodulators or neurotransmitters. The transmitter substances have many subtypes, and interact with each other in complex and varied ways. Depending upon their actions in different parts of the brain, these substances may have many different effects, stimulating neurons in one part of the brain and inhibiting them in another part.

By interfering at different points in the transmission of information in the CNS, psychoactive compounds often may enhance, mimic, or block the effects of transmitter substances. Transmitter substances frequently stimulate or inhibit neurons containing other transmitter substances, which then go on to stimulate or inhibit still more neurons, causing a cascade of events in the CNS which, in the end, leads to a change in emotional state.

Terms Used in the Study of Drugs

Comparisons of how drugs bind to receptors are frequently used to study and describe the properties of unknown drugs. It is important to understand the terms "agonist" and "antagonist," which are used when comparing a drug with unknown properties to a similar drug that is already well-characterized.

Agonist: A drug or chemical compound that binds to the same receptor as the drug under study and exerts similar physiological and psychological effects.

Antagonist: A drug or chemical compound that displaces (competes) at the same receptor as the drug under study, which leads to a decrease in the drug's physiological and psychological effects.

Partial agonist: A drug that has intermediate activity to the drug under study are termed *partial agonists*.

Inverse agonist: A drug that has the opposite effect to the drug under study.

The Biogenic Amine Hypothesis

In the 1950's, researchers observed that reserpine, a drug used to treat hypertension, was causing depressive symptoms in about 15% of the patients taking it. It was hypothesized that taking reserpine leads to a depletion of NE and 5-HT in the CNS by first causing the release, and then preventing the reuptake, of these transmitters from the neuron's storage granules. When not inside storage granules, NE and 5-HT are broken down by the enzyme monoamine oxidase (MAO), leading to a depletion of NE and 5-HT. It was hypothesized that this depletion caused depression.

In the 1960's, as a result of these ideas, Joseph Schildkraut at Harvard University posited the theory that clinical depression was associated with a deficiency of catecholamines (specifically NE) in certain brain regions, and that mania was associated with an excess of NE. This developed into the biogenic amine hypothesis.[1]

The hypothesis is as follows: NE and 5-HT are synthesized from the amino acids tyrosine and tryptophan, respectively. After the transmitters are synthesized, they are stored in the synaptic granules of the neuron, where they are protected from enzymatic degradation. When the nerve cell fires, NE or 5-HT is released from the storage granules into the cell's synaptic cleft; the NE or 5-HT then interacts with post-synaptic receptors. Depending upon appropriate stimulation or inhibition, the next neuron will either fire or be inhibited. At this point, the NE or 5-HT is either catabolized (broken down) by COMT at the synapse, or taken back up into the pre-synaptic side of the neuron and catabolized by MAO. It was believed that antidepressant medications modified some part or parts of this process, causing some change in the neurotransmitter system leading to a change in mood.[1]

Present understanding

It is now known that this early hypothesis is an extremely simplified version of the complex chemistry of the CNS. Since the 1960's, many substances that act as neuromodulators or neurotransmitters have been, and are continuing to be, discovered. These compounds have many subtypes that regulate various functions and emotional states in different parts of the CNS. The structure of the receptor is also much more complex than was initially imagined; every type of receptor can have a variety of different sites on it, with each site responding to different transmitter substances and drugs. Although current theories of how transmitters are synthesized, stored, released and affect emotions are much more detailed, complex and specific, they all have their origins in the biogenic amine theory.[2]

Recent research has documented that the neurobiological substrate of depression, and the mechanism of action of antidepressants, are even more complex than just alterations at the synapse. Changes in the morphology of neurons, such as atrophy of neurons in the prefrontal cortex or the hypothalamus, or an increase in the number of CNS cortico-releasing factor (CRF) cell bodies, may all play a major role in the development of depression. It has also been hypothesized that changes caused by stress in the glucocorticoid receptors in certain regions of the brain (e.g., the hippocampus) contribute to the depressive symptoms.[2]

It is now clearer how the immune system contributes to the pathophysiology of depression. Some immune-mediated medical illnesses can lead to a behavioral syndrome similar to depression, and patients with a primary depressive illness demonstrate alterations in their cytokine levels (the transmitters that are involved with the transmission of pain).[3] The means by which all these processes affect emotions is an extremely active area of research.

The Stress Hypothesis

The stress hypothesis has been gaining credibility among brain researchers over the biogenic amine hypothesis. It posits that depression is caused when the brain's stress mechanism becomes overactive. When a person is stressed, the hypothalamus produces corticotropin-releasing hormone (CRH) which stimulates the pituitary, triggering the release of glucocorticoids (stress hormones such as cortisol) from the adrenal glands. The presence of these stress hormones leads to a decrease in the factors needed to keep neurons healthy. If the stress is prolonged a shrinking of the hippocampus, a key site in the brain for the action of antidepressant drugs, may result.[4]

This theory is supported by findings that the hippocampus is smaller in people who are chronically depressed. Another supporting factor is that it takes antidepressant medications many weeks to reach their optimal effect, which may indicate that neuronal growth is part of the recovery process.[4]

CHAPTER 2 (TREATMENT OF INSOMNIA & ANXIETY DISORDERS)

Sedative-hypnotic drugs

Most drugs in this class interact in some way with the GABA receptor or the ion channel connected to this receptor. It is thought that the GABA receptor is composed of five subunits. Various drugs in this class may react with different subunits, which could account for the differences in their actions, addictive potentials, and adverse effects. Since GABA is usually inhibitory, activation of the GABA receptor by these compounds usually causes sedation.[2]

Antihistamines for sleep induction

Antihistamines are believed to affect the wake-promoter neurons that project from the hypothalamus to the cerebral cortex. When these neurons are blocked by an antihistamine this pathway is suppressed, leading to sedation. This pathway is distinct from the ascending RAS.[5]

CHAPTER 3 (ALCOHOL: USE & ABUSE)

The proposed mechanism of action for alcohol is complex, affecting many different neurotransmitter systems and regions of the CNS. One factor that complicates understanding is that as alcohol concentration increases, its action in the brain becomes more diffuse and more parts of the brain are affected. Another complication is that the brain's response to alcohol is different depending on whether the exposure to alcohol is acute or chronic. Structural changes in the CNS are seen after chronic exposure to alcohol. Below is a simplified version of the current theory of how alcohol affects the CNS.

1. Alcohol has specific effects on GABA and glutamate receptors.[6,7]
2. GABA and glutamate are responsible for much of the inhibitory and excitatory activity in the CNS.
a) At first, alcohol increases inhibitory action of GABA receptors

and decreases excitatory activity of glutamate receptors.
b) Enhancement of GABA activity is responsible for the sedating effect of alcohol.
c) Decrease in glutamate activity in the hippocampus may be the specific cause of impairment of the ability to form new memories while intoxicated.[8]
d) Effect on the hippocampus accounts for lapses in memory, or in more severe instances, blackouts.
e) Chronic ingestion of alcohol can lead to cell injury and death by making neurons more sensitive to excititoxicity produced by glutamate.[6]
3. Alcohol ingestion causes increased release of DA in reward centers of the brain.[6]
a) Release is probably mediated by GABA neurons that connect to DA neurons in reward centers of the brain, leading to the experience of pleasure.
b) The increase in DA activity only takes place while the alcohol level in the blood is rising, not when the level is constant or falling. Because of this, the drinker in search of this pleasurable experience may be motivated to continue drinking to keep the blood-alcohol level rising.[8]

There is some evidence that there may be a common pathway for the mechanism of action of opioids and alcohol. Acute use of alcohol leads to increased endorphin levels. Opioid receptors in the CNS react differently to the acute or chronic presence of alcohol, which contributes to the differences in mood seen when people who are habituated to alcohol are drinking, as compared with the response of people who drink infrequently.[7]

Disulfiram

Disulfiram/Antabuse inhibits the enzymatic oxidation of acetaldehyde to acetate in the metabolism of alcohol to carbon dioxide (CO_2) and water (H_2O). The inhibition of enzyme activity caused by disulfiram is irreversible (until more enzyme is synthesized).

This blockage of enzymatic activity leads to a buildup of acetaldehyde in the blood. If one drinks while taking disulfiram, a buildup of acetaldehyde will occur, causing unpleasant and toxic effects. The chemical reaction that illustrates the action of disulfiram can be seen below.

alcohol → acetaldehyde → acetone → carbon dioxide + water

disulfiram ↑ blocks here   Figure D1

CHAPTER 4 (TREATMENT OF DEPRESSIVE DISORDERS)

Selective serotonin reuptake inhibitors (SSRIs)

As the name indicates, these drugs prevent the reuptake of 5-HT into the presynaptic space. They seem to do this by inhibiting the 5-HT reuptake transporter molecule. Taking SSRIs such as fluoxytene/Prozac, sertraline HCl/Zoloft, paroxetine/Paxil, venlafaxine HCl/Effexor (with more being developed every day) leads to an increase in 5-HT at the synapse.

There may be a lag time of several weeks before maximal decrease of depressive symptoms is experienced. The reason for the lag is not clear; there is some indication that this may be due to the time it takes for neurons to grow. The mechanism of action for these drugs is complex and not completely understood. Although called SSRIs, they probably also have some affect on NE and, to lesser extent, DA.[2]

Tricyclic & heterocyclic antidepressants (TCAs & HCAs)

Tricyclic and heterocyclic antidepressants act by interfering with the transport of NE and 5-HT back into the presynaptic side of the synaptic cleft, resulting in an increase in NE and 5-HT at the synapse.

Other substances that lead to an increase in 5-HT and NE at the synapse may alleviate symptoms of depression. Taking the amino acid l-tryptophan, a precursor to 5-HT, enhances the effect of antidepressant medications, and for some people is effective as an antidepressant even when taken by itself.

Monoamine oxidase inhibitors (MAOIs)

MAOIs inhibit monoamine oxidase (MAO), an enzyme which normally breaks down the monoamines NE, 5-HT, and DA. This breakdown usually takes place when the transmitter substances have been transported from the synaptic cleft back into the presynaptic nerve cell, but have not yet been stored in the synaptic vesicles. The presence of the MAOIs leads to a decrease in degradation by MAO and an increase in levels of available NE, 5-HT, and DA. With these increased MAO levels, the cell does not have to synthesize new transmitters since the old ones were not broken down. The increased amounts of NE and 5-HT affect a complex series of events, resulting in a lessening of the symptoms of depression.[2]

CHAPTER 5 (TREATMENT OF BIPOLAR DISORDER)

Lithium

There have been millions of prescriptions written for lithium over the last 50 years. Researchers are becoming more certain as to how it exerts its effects, and it remains the first choice for treating bipolar disorder. Lithium promotes neuron growth in brain tissue by depressing a mechanism that normally keeps neurons from growing. This allows neurons to form new connections and grow into unoccupied spaces.[9] Lithium also increases levels of brain-derived neurotrophic factor (BDNF), which has been shown to stimulate neuronal growth.[9]

It has been found that cells exposed to lithium for a week are protected from over-stimulation caused by the presence of large amounts of glutamate; this would normally lead to cell death.[10] The presence of lithium leads to a stabilization of glutamate levels. It has been demonstrated that lithium can both slow down and speed up the glutamate reuptake system. Lithium may limit the influx of calcium into nerve cells, which usually takes place in the presence of glutamate and can lead to cell death. If this hypothesis is correct, then taking lithium may also be helpful in other situations where there is cell death, such as with a cardiovascular accident (stroke), Parkinson's, Alzheimer's, and Huntington's diseases.[11]

Anticonvulsant medications

Most anticonvulsant medications have widespread effects in the CNS. They affect nervous transmission in the limbic system, which leads to their anticonvulsant properties. These drugs demonstrate agonist effects at GABA receptors in the CNS. The agonist effects lead to calming due to an increase of neuronal inhibition at GABA receptors.[12]

CHAPTER 6 (STIMULANTS: USE & ABUSE)

Amphetamines

Amphetamines are known to lead to a decrease in the transport of NE and DA back into the presynaptic terminal. They also inhibit the enzyme MAO. This leads to an increased amount of NE and DA at the synapse. The increased DA at the synapse may be the cause of the paranoid psychosis sometimes seen in chronic amphetamine users. DA has a role in the reward system in the CNS. All processes of addiction have some connection to the DA system.[13]

Drugs for attention deficit disorders

The reason stimulant drugs have a calming effect in people with ADHD is not well-understood. It seems clear that NE has a role in the effects, and it is believed that 5-HT also is involved in the action of the drugs used for this purpose. Recent research suggests involvement of NE and DA transporter mechanisms.[14, 15]

Ondansetron (for amphetamine withdrawal)

Ondansetron diminishes the effects of amphetamine by reducing DA availability in the midbrain, leading to an inability to get high when amphetamines are used.[16]

Cocaine

Taking cocaine leads to a decrease in the transport of NE and DA from the synapse. It has been demonstrated that cocaine strongly binds to the DA reuptake transporter molecule; this prevents reuptake of DA into the presynaptic cells, leading to an increased DA effect at the synapse.[13] Large amounts of DA at the synapse leads to the characteristic euphoria and stimulation (rush) experienced when cocaine is used.

Nicotine

There is evidence that nornicotine, an active metabolite of nicotine and a major alkaloid found in tobacco, increases DA release in the CNS. The nornicotine stimulates nicotinic receptors in the CNS (acts as an agonist at these receptors), which then causes the release of DA.[17]

Caffeine

Caffeine is believed to act as an antagonist to adenosine (an inhibitory neurotransmitter).[18] Blockade of the adenosine receptors leads to stimulation of inhibitory GABA neurons, leading to an increase in DA reward.[19] Caffeine is also known to affect ACh in the cortex, which may be linked to caffeine's ability to increase mental acuity.[20]

CHAPTER 7 (TREATMENT OF PSYCHOTIC DISORDERS)

Antipsychotic drugs

All antipsychotic drugs influence the action and response of the CNS to NE, DA, and 5-HT in varying amounts and in various areas of the brain. These transmitters have many subtypes that are active in different parts of the brain, and have different effects. The areas of the CNS most affected by these medications are the:

- hypothalamus
- basal ganglia
- limbic system
- cerebral cortex[21]

Second generation antipsychotic medications (SGAs)

Some SGAs also affect transmission at histamine, GABA, glutamate, NMDA, and ACh sites.[22] Studies show a relationship between DA and GABA. As DA levels increase, GABA levels decrease. Low levels of GABA are correlated with disorganized thought processes. High levels of DA may suppress GABA, resulting in a thought disorder. The inhibition of neuronal activity due to GABA may be necessary to keep the number of signals in the CNS at a level and frequency that can be received and assimilated in a way that makes sense. The SGAs impact 5-HT transmission to a greater extent than do the traditional antipsychotics.[23]

Dopamine system stabilizers (DSSs)

The new DSSs act as partial DA agonists.[24] They increase DA transmission in some parts of the brain (frontal lobes) where it is believed DA is too low; this increase helps with the negative symptoms of schizophrenia. DSSs decrease DA transmission in other parts of the CNS (limbic system) where it is thought the DA levels are too high; this decrease helps alleviate the positive symptoms of schizophrenia.[25]

CHAPTER 8 (PAIN & TREATMENTS OF PAIN)

Pain medications

One way opioids exert their effect is by decreasing neuronal activity by selectively binding to specific opioid receptors in the CNS. Many of these opioid sites are in the hypothalamus. Large numbers of opioid receptors are also found outside of the CNS in the intestine, where opioids act as antidiarrhea agents by slowing peristalsis. The compound paregoric acts in this way, and is often given to children with severe diarrhea. Opioids also act as neuromodulators and inhibit the release of Substance P, DA, and ACh, leading to a decrease in the transmission of the pain impulse.[26]

Nonsteroidal anti-inflammatory agents (NSAIDs)

One site where NSAIDs are believed to act is at the glycine receptors in the spinal cord. The NSAIDs block prostaglandin production, which prevents the inhibitory action of the prostaglandins on the glycine receptors. When the glycine receptors are inhibited, pain signals are transmitted to the brain.[27]

Morphine & the endorphins

Morphine and related compounds exert their analgesic and other actions by interacting with specific opioid receptors. The specificity of these receptors led investigators to postulate the existence of an endogenous (internally generated) substance in the CNS that is analogous to the opioids.

These endogenous substances have been named endorphins, for "endogenous morphine-like substances." The first endorphins to be characterized were named enkephalins; these were found to be only mildly analgesic, but to have a high addictive potential. It is believed that enkephalins are inhibitory neurotransmitters. Chronic use of opioids leads to a decrease in the production of endogenous enkephalins and endorphins.

The opioid receptors, which were previously called delta, kappa, and mu, have been reclassified by a subcommittee of the International Union of Pharmacology as OP1 (delta), OP2 (kappa), and OP3 (mu).

Their properties are:

OP1 receptors: These mediate analgesia, sedation, and possibly the release of some hormones.

OP2 receptors: These are responsible for analgesia, dysphoria and some psychotomimetic effects (e.g., disorientation and/or depersonalization), and sedation.

OP3 receptors: These are responsible for analgesia, euphoria, respiratory depression, and meiosis (a type of cell division).

Buprenorphine

This drug acts on OP3 receptors to cause analgesia, euphoria, and other opioid effects. It is a partial agonist to diacetylmorphine/heroin, but less potent. It binds strongly to the OP3 receptor, preventing any euphoria if other opioids are used. It is long-acting, which can make the detox process more gentle. For those who have been heavy drug users it can trigger withdrawal symptoms.[28]

CHAPTER 9 (CONSCIOUSNESS-ALERTING DRUGS)

Dimethyltryptamine (DMT) & ayahuasca

DMT, either by itself or in ayahuasca, exerts its effects by acting as an antagonist at 5-HT receptors.[29] Ayahuasca also contains an MAO inhibitor which, by preventing enzymatic degradation by MAO, allows for absorption of the DMT and prolongs its activity.[30]

Lysergic Acid Diethylamide (LSD, "acid")

LSD is in a group of compounds called indolealkylamines. One of its properties is that it resembles 5-HT in chemical structure; it may act as a 5-HT agonist. It also has some effect at the NE receptors. The specific mechanism of action of LSD remains unclear.

Marijuana & hashish

There are endogenous substances called endocannabinoids (e.g., anandamide) in the CNS. These bind to specific cannabinoid receptors and act as retrograde messengers in the brain. These compounds are fat-soluble and cannot be easily contained in vesicles. Synthesis and release of the endocannabinoids is due to postsynaptic depolarization. The endocannabinoids bind to presynaptic receptors. Inactivation of the endocannabinoids is probably due to an enzyme that specifically degrades this class of lipids (fats).[31] Recent research indicates that the endogenous cannabinoid system, which is activated by THC, protects neurons against cell death after brain trauma.[32]

MDMA ("ecstasy")

MDMA causes the release of, and a decrease in, reuptake of 5-HT. It also binds to the receptors for other neurotransmitters, leading to its other effects (e.g., hallucinations, hypertension). It is thought that DA is involved in the pleasurable effects of MDMA.[33]

Phencyclidine (PCP) & Ketamine

PCP and Ketamine block (act as antagonists) at the N-methyl-D-aspartate (NMDA) receptors. This blocking of the receptors may cause analgesia by reducing the capacity of neuronal projections to conduct and coordinate signals. It is believed that this process also takes place in "near death" experiences. Phencyclidine and Ketamine may cause cell death in some neurons.[34]

Phencyclidine is known to induce psychotic episodes in normal subjects, and to exacerbate psychosis in schizophrenics. Phencyclidine and Ketamine appear to enhance glutamate transmission at non-NMDA receptors. This may lead to a disorganization of cortical activity (as is found in schizophrenia).[35, 36] The brain regions that appear to play a role in the pathophysiology of schizophrenia (prefrontal cortex, hippocampus, basal ganglia) are the areas most likely involved in the psychotomimetic action of phencyclidine.[34, 36]

Peyote

As with most botanicals, there are many chemical compounds present in the cactus *Lophophora williamsii* that might cause the symptoms of intoxication. There are 32 alkaloids in peyote, most of which are in the phenylethylamine category; many of these may have psychedelic activity. The most widely studied is mescaline, which resembles DA, NE, and the amphetamines in its chemical structure. The specific mechanism of action remains unclear.

Psilocybin

The active ingredient in psilocybin is 4, hydroxymethyltryptamine.

This molecule is similar to 5-HT and tryptophan (a 5-HT precursor). Because of this similarity, it is believed to act at the 5-HT receptors.[37]

CHAPTER 10 (COGNITION-ENHANCING DRUGS)

Some cholinergic drugs

These drugs affect the ACh system in the CNS and seem to work in conjunction with the steroid hormones. It has been demonstrated that when the adrenal glands have been removed, this type of drug has no effect. ACh levels decrease with age. This decrease may be one factor that leads to the loss of cognitive functioning which is often seen with aging. Nootropic drugs act synergistically when taken in combination with other nootropics.[35]

Ampakines

The group of drugs called ampakines activate AMPA-type receptors. Through this activation they enhance glutamate transmission in the CNS. It is believed that this enhancement may help to improve cognitive abilities.[38]

References for Appendix D

1. Schildkraut, J. J. (1965). The catecholamine hypothesis of affective disorders: A review of supporting evidence. *Am. J. Psychiatry,* 122, 509.
2. Bloom, F. E. & Kupfer, D. J. (Eds.) (1995). *Psychopharmacology: The fourth generation of progress.* New York: Raven Press.
3. Dunn, A. J. & Wang, J. (1995). Cytokine effects on CNS biogenic amines. *Neuroimmunomodulation,* 2, 319.
4. Leonard, B. (2000). Stress, depression and the activation of the immune system. *World J. Biol. Psychiatry,* 1(1), 17–25.
5. Stahl, S. M. (2002). Awakening to the psychopharmacology of sleep and arousal: Novel neurotransmitters and wake-promoting drugs. *J. Clinical Psychiatry,* 63(4), 339–402.
6. Tabakoff, B. & Hoffman, P. L. (1993). The neurochemistry of alcohol. *Current Opinion in Psychiatry,* 6, 388–394.
7. Bonner, A. B. (1994). Biological mechanisms of alcohol dependence. *Current Opinion in Psychiatry,* 7, 262–268.
8. Kuhn, C., Schwartzwelder, S. & Wilson, W. (1998). *BUZZED: The straight facts*

about the most used and abused drugs from alcohol to ecstasy. New York: W. W. Norton and Co.

9. Medina, J., PHD. (2003). Intracellular signaling and mood stabilizers. *Psychiatric Times,* XX(12), 32–36.

10. Nonaka, S., Hough, C. J., & Chuang, D. (1998). Chronic lithium treatment robustly protects neurons in the central nervous system against excitotoxicity by inhibiting N-methyl-D-aspartate receptor-mediated calcium influx. *Proceedings of the National Academy of Sciences,* March 3, 95, 2641–2647.

11. Dixon, J. F. & Hokin, L. E. (1988). Lithium acutely inhibits and chronically up-regulates and stabilizes glutamate uptake by presynaptic nerve endings in mouse cerebral cortex. *Proceedings of the National Academy of Sciences,* July 7, 95(14), 8363–8368.

12. Pope, H. G. Jr., Mc Elroy, S. L., Keck, P. E. Jr. & Hudson, J. I. (1991). Valproate in the treatment of acute mania: A placebo controlled study. *Arch. Gen. Psychiatry,* 48, 62–68.

13. Schuckit, M. A. (1997). Science, medicine, and the future: Substance use disorders. *BMJ,* 314, 1605–1608.

14. MacMaster, F. P., Carrey, N., Sparkes, S. & Kusumakar, V. (2002). Proton spectroscopy in medication-free pediatric attention deficit/hyperactivity disorder: A preliminary case series. *J. Child Adolescent Psychopharm.,* Winter, 12, 331–336.

15. Gainetdinov, R. R., Wetsel, W. C., Jones, S. R., Levin, E. D., Jaber, & M., Caron, M. G. R. (1999). Role of serotonin in the paradoxical calming effect of psychostimulants on hyperactivity. *Science,* 283(5400), 397–401.

16. Johnson, B. A. (2000). Ondansetron for reduction of drinking among biologically predisposed alcoholic patients. *JAMA,* 284(8), 36.

17. Teng, L., Crooks, P. A., Buckston, S. T. & Dwoskin, L. P. (1997). Nicotinic-receptor mediation of S(-)nornicotine-evoked [^{3}H] overflow from rat striatal slices preloaded with [^{3}H] dopamine. *Psychopharm. Exp. Ther.,* 283(2), 778–787.

18. Kaplan, G. B., Greenblatt, D. J., Kent, M. A., Cotreau, M. M., Arcelin, G. & Shader, R. I. (1992). Caffeine-induced behavioral stimulation is dose-dependent and associated with A1 adenosine receptor occupancy. *Neuropsychopharm.,* 6, 145–153.

19. Daly, J. W. & Fredholm, B. B. (1998). Caffeine-an atypical drug of dependence. *Drug and Alcohol Dependence,* 51, 199–206.

20. Acquas, E., PHD, Gianluigi, T., PHD & Di Chiara, G. (2002). Differential effects of caffeine on dopamine and acetylcholine transmission in brain areas of drug-naive and caffeine-pretreated rats. *Neuropsychopharm.,* 27, 182–193.

21. Hyman, Steven E., MD. (1988). Recent developments in neurobiology: Part 1. Synaptic transmission. *Psychosomatics,* 29, 2.

22. Singh, A. N., Barlas, C., Singh, S., Franks, P. & Mishra, R. K. (1996). A neurochemical basis for the antipsychotic activity of loxapine: Interactions with dopamine D1, D2, D4 and serotonin 5-HT2 receptor subtypes. *J. Psychiatry Neurosci.,* 21(1), 29–35.

23. Kaplan, H. I. & Sadock, B. J. Eds. (1995). *Comprehensive Textbook of Psychiatry.*

Baltimore: Williams and Wilkins.

24. Tandon, R. (2002). New steps in the evolution of antipsychotics: The role of partial agonists. *US Psych. Congress*, October, Las Vegas, NV.

25. Stahl, S. M. (2001). Dopamine system stabilizers, aripiprazole, and the next generation of antipsychotics, Part I: "Goldilocks" actions at dopamine receptors, and Part II: Illustrating their mechanisms of action. *J. Clinical Psychiatry*, 62(11), 841–842 and 62(12), 923–924.

26. Mantyh, P. (2000). Understanding substance P and the substance P receptor. Presented at the XXIInd Congress of the Collegium Internationale Neuro-Psychopharmacologicum (CINP); July 10, Brussels, Belgium. Abstract.

27. Marx, J. (2004). Locating a new step in pain's pathway. *Science,* 304, 811.

28. Fingerhood, M. I., Thompson, M. R. & Jasinski, D. R. (2001). A comparison of clonidine and buprenorphine in the outpatient treatment of opiate withdrawal. *Substance Abuse*, 22(3), 193–199.

29. Pierce, P. A. & Peroutka, S. J. (1989). Hallucinogenic drug interactions with neurotransmitter receptor binding sites in human cortex. *Psychopharm.*, 97, 118–122.

30. Callaway, J. C., McKenna, D. J., Grob, C. S., Brito, G. S., Raymon, L. P., Poland, R. E., Andrade, E. N., Andrade, E. O. & Mash, D. C. (1999). Pharmacokinetics of *hoasca* alkaloids in healthy humans. *J. Ethnopharmacol.,* 65, 243–256.

31. Bracey, M. H., Hanson, M. A., Masuda, K. R., Stevens, R. C. & Cravatt, B. F. (2002). Structural adaptations in a membrane enzyme that terminates endocannabinoid signaling. *Science,* 298, 1793–1796.

32. Mechoulam, R. & Lichtman, A. H. (2003). Stout guards of the central nervous system. *Science,* 302, 65, 67.

33. Solowij, N. (1993). Ecstasy (3,4-methylenedioxymethamphetamine). *Current Opinion in Psychiatry*, 6, 411–415.

34. Jansen, K. L. R. (1996) Using ketamine to induce the near-death experience: Mechanism of action and therapeutic potential. *Yearbook for Ethnomedicine and the Study of Consciousness* (Jahrbuch fur Ethnomedizin und Bewubtseinsforschung), Issue 4, 1995. C. Ratsch; J. R. Baker (Eds.), VWB, Berlin, pp. 55–81.

35. Moghaddam, B. (2003). Glutamate and disorders of cognition and motivation, April 13–15, *New York Academy of Sciences.*

36. O'Donnell, P. & Grace, A. A. (1998). Phencyclidine interferes with the hippocampal gating of nucleus accumbens neuronal activity in vivo. *Neuroscience*, 87(4), 823–830.

37. Vollenweider, F. X., Vontobel, P., Hell, D. & Leenders, K. L. (1999). 5-HT modulation of dopamine release in basal ganglia in psilocybin-induced psychosis in man—A PET study with [¹¹C] raclopride. *Neuropsychopharm.*, 20(5), 424–433.

38. Berry-Kravis, E., MD, Hagerman, R. J., MD & Cook E., MD. (2002). New drug that enhances glutamate transmission in the brain being evaluated for Fragile X. *Science Daily Magazine.* Retrieved Oct. 22, 2003 from http://www.rush.edu/

Appendix E
Other Types of Drug Responses

TOLERANCE

In pharmacological terms, "tolerance" means a decrease in a person's response to a drug; an increase in dosage becomes necessary to obtain the desired effect.[1] Tolerances to different effects of a drug develop at different rates. As an example, a particular sedative may induce sleep, cause euphoria, and inhibit psychomotor performance. Since tolerance to the psychomotor effect develops more slowly than tolerance to the euphoric effect, a person might increase the dosage of a sedative drug to obtain a desired amount of euphoria while not realizing that this increase may result in a dangerous impairment of the ability to drive a car.

Enzymatic tolerance

Also known as dispositional tolerance, this is due to an increase in the production of liver enzymes that are synthesized to metabolize a drug. The rate at which the drug is metabolized increases as tolerance develops. The more rapid metabolism can lead to taking higher doses of the drug to maintain a desired effect. The body's response to the use of barbiturates is an example of this type of tolerance.[1]

Cellular or pharmacodynamic tolerance

This type of tolerance occurs when the target cell or receptor for the drug changes over time due to exposure to the drug. When this occurs, more drug is required to produce a desired effect, a phenomenon known as "down regulation" of the receptors. Using amphetamines causes this type of tolerance.[1]

Cross-tolerance

This is a type of cellular tolerance that occurs when tolerance develops to drugs in the same class, or in similar classes, due to a change in the receptor for those drugs. An example is the cross-tolerance that develops between the use of opioids and other types of narcotics. A person taking one type of pain killer may develop a tolerance to others, even when the drugs are completely different in their chemical structures.[2]

Note: Any drug may cause the development of any or all of the different types of tolerances.

PHYSICAL DEPENDENCE, ADDICTION, & ABUSE

Physical dependence

Physical dependence has been defined in many different ways. One definition states that physical dependence occurs when a person who has been taking a particular drug on a regular basis begins to require that drug to function normally, experiences withdrawal symptoms with abstinence, and is able to terminate the withdrawal symptoms by taking the drug. It sometimes difficult to clearly delineate between physical and psychological symptoms of withdrawal.

The *DSM-IV* states that dependence involves the impaired control of psychoactive substance use and continued use despite adverse consequences. It includes legal, illegal, and prescription drugs on its list of drugs that have a potential for substance dependence. Alcohol, amphetamines, antianxiety drugs, cannabis, cocaine, hallucinogens, nicotine, and sedatives are a few of the drugs of potential abuse listed in the *DSM-IV*.[3]

In this book the term "physical dependence" is used to denote a state of physiological need for a drug. In other words, if the drug is not taken, physical withdrawal symptoms will be experienced. Physical dependence is not meant to signify that a drug is being used in an addictive or abusive manner.

Addiction

In this book the term "addiction" is used when taking a drug leads to some destructive consequence in a person's life. The amount or frequency of drug use is not the determining factor. For example, someone can be a binge drinker and consume alcohol only once a year, but if there are negative consequences to that drinking episode the use is considered an addiction.

Abuse

The term "abuse" in the *DSM-IV* indicates maladaptive patterns of psychoactive substance use. This category includes substance use in situations that may be physically hazardous, such as while driving. It also includes continued use despite knowledge that a social, psychological, occupational, or physical problem is being caused by use of the psychoactive substance. According to the *DSM-IV*, the symptoms must have persisted for at least one month.[3]

WITHDRAWAL

Withdrawal is a syndrome of autonomic dysfunction that occurs when someone who has become physically dependent on a drug stops taking it. Withdrawal symptoms may or may not be the same as those of the original disorder for which the medication was taken. For many drugs, withdrawal symptoms are the opposite of the drug's usual effects. For example, if a drug is taken to decrease anxiety (typically a BZ), anxiety and agitation will increase when the drug is withdrawn.[1]

ALLERGIC REACTIONS

Another common type of response to a drug is an allergic reaction. This type of reaction involves the immune system. One person's immune system may react violently to a substance or drug that is harmless to the general population. Specifically, in an allergic reaction an antibody (usually immunoglobulin E) will bind to an allergen (the drug) and to a mast cell containing heparin (an anticoagulant) and histamine, or to a basophil (a type of white blood cell). This process signals a release of histamine and other chemicals into the bloodstream. The release of these substances causes swelling, heat, and itching.[4]

A classical allergic reaction is defined very specifically. This type of reaction is very serious and can be fatal. Often, the first sign of an allergic reaction is the development of a skin rash. If a rash develops while someone is taking medication, the prescribing physician should be notified immediately. It is likely that the physician will advise that the drug be discontinued and never taken again. The physician must be informed of any drug allergies. Many drugs are chemically similar, and an allergy to one drug may serve as a warning of a possible allergic reaction to others in the same chemical class.[4]

Allergies, intolerances, & sensitivities

The term "allergy" is now being used more broadly to include what in the past had been called the "intolerances" or "sensitivities" that some people have to milk, wheat, or other foods. Digestive problems and headaches are the usual symptoms seen with these food intolerances or sensitivities. One cause can be an absence of the enzyme necessary to digest the specific food properly, e.g., lactose intolerance.

It is also possible for a person to have a true allergic reaction to a food or a food group. Well-known examples of this are allergies to shellfish or peanuts. The symptoms of this type of food allergy usually include burning of the lips or mouth, skin rash, severe cramping, and diarrhea. If a food allergy is suspected, one should not consume the suspect food and consult a physician. This type of classical allergy can be fatal.[4]

PLACEBO EFFECTS

A placebo is defined as a substance that contains no known pharmacologically-active ingredient, yet elicits a therapeutic response. The specific mechanism for this type of response is not yet understood, but it is thought to be due mainly to the patient's expectations. The standard finding is that a placebo is effective in about 33% of the people to whom it is administered. When new drugs are developed, it is important to keep in mind that usually a response rate much higher than the response to a placebo needs to occur for the drug to be considered pharmacologically active.

This standard for therapeutic effectiveness is influenced by many factors, including the seriousness of the disease the drug is designed to treat, the potential adverse effects or lack of adverse effects from the drug, and the availability of alternative treatments or medications.

References for Appendix E

1. Chiang, W. K., MD & Goldfrank, L. R., MD. (1990). Substance withdrawal. *Emergency Medicine Clinics of North America,* Aug., 8(3), 613–614.
2. Julian, Robert, MD, PhD. (1995). *A primer of drug action* (7th ed.). New York: W. H. Freeman & Co.
3. American Psychiatric Association. (1994). *Diagnostic and statistical manual of mental disorders* (4th ed.). Washington, DC: American Psychiatric Association.
4. *The Merck manual of diagnosis and therapy* (17th ed.). (2001). Rahway, NJ: Merck Sharp & Dohme Research Laboratories.

Final Thoughts

New psychoactive medications are constantly being developed. It is neither practical, nor necessary, for the psychotherapist to study the mechanisms of actions of these drugs, or learn details such as which neurotransmitters are affected. If a client is taking medication, what is important is that the therapist know the class of drug being taken and recognize whether it is an appropriate treatment for the presenting symptoms. It is also vital that the therapist be able to:

- assess whether a client might benefit from the use of psychoactive medication
- discuss the use of psychoactive medication in a knowledgeable and unbiased way
- work collegially with prescribing psychiatrists

With the increased use of psychoactive medications, these skills are prerequisites for all psychotherapists.

Common Psychiatric Medications & Nonprescription Drugs

Sedative-Hypnotic & Antianxiety Medications

Generic name/Brand name ®	Avg. daily dose (mg)

Benzodiazepines (BZs)

alprazolam/Xanax	0.25–8
clorazepate/Tranxene	3.75–15
chlordiazepoxide/Librium	5–250
clonazepam/Klonopin	1–6
diazepam/Valium	2–40
flurazepam/Dalmane	15–60
lorazepam/Ativan	0.5–1
oxazepam/Serax	30–120
triazolam/Halcion	0.25–0.5
prazepam/Centrax	20–60
temazepam/Restoril	15–30

Atypical Hypnotics

estazolam/ProSom	1–2
sodium oxybate/Xyrem	4.5–9 (grams)
zaleplon/Sonata	5–20
zolpidem/Ambien	5–10

Other Medications for Anxiety

atenolol/Tenormin	25–100
buspirone/BuSpar	15–60
clonidine/Catapres	0.1–3
escitalopram/Lexapro	10
hydroxyzine/Atarax/Vistaril	50–400
melatonin	0.3–3
propanolol/Inderal	80–640

Opioids & Pain Medications

buprenorphine/Subutex	16
buprenorphine + naloxone/Suboxone	4–24
butorphanol/Stadol (i.m. or i.v.)	12–48
codeine	45–240
dezocine/Dalgan (i.m. or s.c.)	6–12
diacetylmorphine (heroin)	—
fentanyl/Actiq (transmucosal)/ Duragesic/Sublimaze (transdermal)	varies
hydrocodone/Vicodin	7.5–30
hydromorphone/Dilaudid	1 & up
meperidine/Demerol (i.m.)	200–7500
methadone/Dolophine	10–80
morphine (i.m.)	10–30
nalbuphine/Nubain	10–160
oxycodone/OxyContin	20–320
oxymorphone/Numorphan (i.m. or s.c.)	4–6
pentazocine/Talwin	22.5–30
propoxyphene/Darvon	195–390

Nootropic Medications

donepezil/Aricept	5–10
galantamine/Reminyl	16–24
memantine/Namenda	20
rivastigmine/Exelon	3–12
tacrine/Cognex	40–80

Bipolar Disorder Medications

lithium/Eskalith/Lithobid	600–2400
lamotrigine/Lamictal	50–500
olanzapine+fluoxetine/Symbyax	6/25–12/50
risperidone/Risperdal	4–16

Anticonvulsants for Mania

carbamazepine/Tegretol	600–1600
gabapentin/Neurontin	900–1800
oxcarbazepine/Trileptal	300–1200
tiagabine/Gabitril	4–56
topiramate/Topamax	25–400
valproate/Depakene/Depakote	750

Central Nervous System (CNS) Stimulants

atomoxetine/Strattera	40–80
caffeine	—
cocaine	—
dextroamphetamine/ Dexedrine	5–40
dextroamphetamine; amphetamine/Adderall	2.5–40
methamphetamine/Methedrine/Desoxyn	5–25
methylphenidate/Ritalin/Concerta	5–50
modafinil/Provigil	100–200
nicotine	—

Antipsychotic Medications

First Generation Antipsychotics (FGAs)

chlorpromazine/Thorazine	50–1500
fluphenazine/Prolixin	3–45
haloperidol/Haldol	2–40
loxapine/Loxitane	50–225
molindone/Moban	20–225
perphenazine/Trilafon	8–60
thioridazine/Mellaril	150–800

Second Generation Antipsychotics (SGAs)

clozapine/Clozaril	300–900
olanzapine/Zyprexa/Zydiss (soluble on tongue)	5–20
quetiapine/Seroquel	25–400
risperidone/Risperdal/Consta (i.m.)	4–16
ziprasidone/Geodon	40–160

Dopamine System Stabilizers (DSSs)

aripiprazole/Abilify	10–15

DOSES ARE ORAL UNLESS INDICATED.

THIS IS NOT A COMPLETE LIST.

SEE WWW.RXLIST.COM FOR UP-TO-DATE INFORMATION ON PRESCRIPTION DRUGS.

Drugs & Clients

What Every Psychotherapist Needs to Know
by Padma Catell, PhD

www.drugsandclients.com

Antidepressant Medications

Tricyclic & Heterocyclic Antidepressants (TCAs & HCAs)

amitriptyline/Elavil	50–300
desipramine/Norpramin	100–300
doxepin/Sinequan/Adapin	100–300
imipramine/Tofranil	25–300
maprotiline/Ludiomil	150–225
nortriptyline/Aventyl/Pamelor	50–150
protriptyline/Vivactil	20–60

Atypical Antidepressants

amoxapine/Asendin	150–400
aprepitant/Emend	not yet available
bupropion/Wellbutrin/Zyban	200–450
mirtazapine/Remeron	15–45
trazadone/Desyrel	200–400

Selective Serotonin Reuptake Inhibitors (SSRIs)

citalopram/Celexa	10–60
clomipramine/Anafranil	25–250
escitalopram/Lexapro	10
fluoxetine/Prozac	10–80
fluvoxamine/Luvox	50–300
paroxetine/Paxil	10–60
sertraline/Zoloft	25–200
venlafaxine/Effexor (an SNRI at higher doses)	75–375

Monoamine Oxidase Inhibitors (MAOIs)

isocarboxazid/Marplan	10–60
phenelzine/Nardil	30–90
tranylcypromine/Parnate	20–60
selegiline/Eldepryl (transdermal)	5–20

Misc. Medications

benztropine/Cogentin	150–250
disulfiram/Antabuse	125–500
nalmefene/Revex	varies
naloxone/Narcan (i.v.)	.04–2
naltrexone/Trexan/ReVia	25–150
nizatidine/Axid	75–300
ondansetron/Zofran	4–300
sildenafil/Viagra	25–100
yohimbine/Actibine/Yocon/Yohimex	2.5–16

Other Treatments for Dementia

ampakines (may improve cognition)

antiamyloid treatments (gene therapy or vaccines)

antioxidants

COX-2 inhibitors (anti-inflammatory agents)

ginkgo (increases blood flow to CNS)

hormone replacement therapy (estrogens or androgens)

huperzine/HupA (ACh esterase inhibitor)

neurotropic agents (human nerve growth factor)

nicotine (stimulates ACh)

NSAIDs (nonsteroidal anti-inflammatory drugs)

phosphotidylserine/PtdSer (natural fat-soluble nutrient)

selegiline/Eldepryl (MAO inhibitor)

statin drugs (lower cholesterol)

vitamin C (antioxidant)

vitamin E (antioxidant)

Index

O

Olanzapine (Zyprexa), 56, 72, 86, 97t., 104, 106, 107, 209t.
  (Zydiss, soluble on tongue), 97t., 209t.
Older adults:
  Alzheimer's disease, 148–150
  caffeine effects, 83
  changing sleep patterns, 2, 14
Omega-3 fatty acids, 159
Ondansetron (Zofran), 209t.
  use in alcohol withdrawal, 40
  use in amphetamine withdrawal, 77
  mechanism of action, 194
  treatment of tardive dyskinesia, 101
Opioids, 114–122. *See also* endorphins
  addiction, 117
  adverse effects (*See also* by drug), 115
  analgesic implants, 122
  antagonist, 39, 117, 118, 122
  mechanism of action, 196, 197
  by name:
    codeine, 114t.
    heroin, 120, 143
    methadone, 114, 114t., 120–121
    morphine, 111, 114t., 116, 197
    opium, 114
    oxycodone (Percodan), 114t.
    oxycodone HCl (Oxycontin), 114t., 122
    oxycodone + naltrexone (Oxytrex), 122
    oxymorphone (Numorphan), 114t.
  nerve-cell-destroying toxins, 123
  neuropeptides, 182
  overdose, 116, 117–118

receptors, 39, 115, 120, 182, 191, 197
  time-line for withdrawal, 119t.
  withdrawal and addiction treatment, 118–122
    buprenorphine, 121, 208t.
    clonidine, 29t., 87, 120, 208t.
    methadone maintenance, 120–121
    nalmefene, 117, 118, 209t.
    naloxone, 117, 118, 121, 209t.
    Rapid Detox, 121–122
Opium, 111, 114, 145. *See also* opioids
Orange, 166t.
Orexin, 7, 182. *See also* hypocretin
Osmond, Humphrey, 127
"Out-of-body" experiences, 141, 143
Oxazepam (Serax), 22t., 208t.
Oxcarbazepine (Trileptal), 70, 208t.
Oxycodone HCl, 114t., 122, 208t.
Oxycontin. *See* oxycodone HCl

P

Pain, 57, 78, 82, 111–124, 141, 156, 166t., 182–183, 189
  benzodiazepines and memory of, 25
  chronic, 113, 115, 122, 123, 124
  hierarchy in treatment of, 112–113
  serotonin and, 111
Pain medications, 111, 115, 122–124, *See also* opioids
  addiction to, 117
  adverse effects, 115
  anticonvulsants, 113
  antidepressants, 111–112, 113
  benzodiazepines, 113–114
  Brompton's cocktail, 78
  dorsal root surgery, 123

About the Author

Padma Catell, Ph.D., is an Associate Professor of Psychology at the California Institute of Integral Studies, a licensed Psychologist, and a Marriage and Family Therapist. She also earned a B.A. in Biology from Hunter College and an M.A. in Biology from the City University of New York with a specialization in pharmacology, which she studied at the Mount Sinai School of Medicine. She has been teaching psychopharmacology at CIIS and other graduate schools in the San Francisco 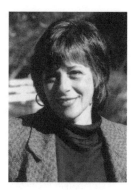 Bay area since 1984. Her advanced degrees in both Biology and Psychology, combined with her extensive teaching and clinical experience, make Dr. Catell uniquely qualified to understand and address the problems facing today's psychotherapists in this rapidly changing, highly controversial, and increasingly important area of psychology.

Psychopharmacology for Psychotherapists

Drugs and Clients is for all therapists, health-care professionals, and graduate students who are not trained in the specialty of psychiatry — $39.95.

Reference Card Set. Two tables from the book, pps. 166 and 208–209, enlarged and printed on sturdy 8.5" X 11" card stock — $9.95 per set.

Free Reference Card Set & Free Shipping! Receive a free reference card set and free shipping with each book purchased directly from us.

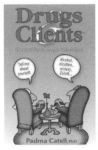

Drugs & Clients
only $39.95
ISBN: 092915076-7

Reference Card Set
Two 8.5 X 11" cards — only $9.95
• Common Psychiatric Medications
• Psychological Uses of Essential Oils

www.drugsandclients.com
FAX: 707-778-0880 • PHONE: 800-752-7730

SEND CHECKS OR MONEY ORDERS (NO CASH) TO:
Solarium Press P.O. Box 2503, Petaluma, CA 94953